ISBN 979-8-218-38946-8 (Hardcover)

Library of Congress Control Number: 2024904805

Front and back cover image by Kaitlin Walsh
Book design by Kaitlin Walsh

Printed and bound in Canada
First printing April 2024

Published by Lyon Road Art
1100 Frank H Street
Waunakee, WI 53597

www.lyonroadart.com

Dedicated to Henry, Rosie and Tommy.
Thank you for your patience
while I wrote my "pooms."

And to Papa Bruce,
thank you for lighting the fire.

PREFACE

My grandpa has a gift for turning knowledge into entertainment. He has a savant-like memory, and would use his stockpiled anecdotes to recite history, weave stories and, my favorite, create mini dinner-table trivia games for my siblings and me throughout our childhood. The best part was that if we got our question right, he'd give us a nickel—a whole nickel!—for our subject mastery. History was probably his favorite topic, but mine was hands-down anatomy. As a retired dentist, he had an arsenal of juicy anatomical factoids that fed my hungry brain like candy. My younger siblings would get the easy questions—"where are the smallest bones in the body?" (the ear, I knew, and it was a physical strain to keep my mouth shut); my older brother and I would get the hard ones—"what are their names in Latin, and what do they mean in English?" (incus, malleus and stapes; anvil, hammer and stirrup).

The thrill of the game was partly why these evenings spoke to me. Receiving accolades and approval from my beloved papa, and later showing off an eight-year old's grasp of Latin terminology to impressed adults, filled me with a delicious pride. But my reaction went deeper. My grandpa's handling of the subject, treating organs and bones and cells and structures as peculiar, poignant and clever characters in life's most fascinating play, implanted in me an eternal reverence for our inner workings.

Take, for example, his story about a small structure on the sphenoid, the skull bone that rests below the brain. Perched atop this delicate, butterfly-like bone is the sella turcica, which is Latin for "Turkish saddle", and exactly what the little formation resembles. Cradled in this saddle is the illustrious pituitary gland, gracefully suspended from the hypothalamus above. What imagery! What poetry! Countless such narratives woven into my childhood begins to explain the depth and longevity of my fascination with anatomy.

Perhaps this interest would have faded if I hadn't later been exposed to teachers who approached instruction the same way my grandpa did. In high school, a new anatomy teacher came bounding into my life. Well-known in the school for his wild stories (he chose to have his teeth pulled with no anesthesia!) and his exuberant personality (on reproductive anatomy day, he ran around the room, impersonating the frenetic energy of a spermatozoa!), he oozed excitement for the subject. I had been getting more invested in art over the years, but his course reinvigorated a desire to include anatomy as a part of my career.

These dual passions eventually led me to the field of medical illustration. After finishing all the disparate prerequisites, I entered a biomedical visualization graduate program at the University of Illinois at Chicago. My anatomy professors there had it too, "it" being that fizzing zeal for anatomy. I recall one PT instructor hinting for days about the upcoming "story of the lumbricals", where we'd learn how they extend *and* flex two joints *at the same time*, as though it was a big movie that was about to premiere, and we were lucky enough to have tickets. Or my lab professor getting so excited about what he was showing us that he did not notice, or perhaps didn't care, that his glove had ripped and he was digging bare-handed through cadaver fat to find an elusive nerve with the same fervor my dog has for buried sticks. Gross, yes, but his enthusiasm was infectious and endearing.

It's that enthusiasm, that love of a subject, that nestled its way into my heart, sparking a long-burning fire that I eventually stoked into a career. From these teachers I realized that the elements of a good story can be found in the most unexpected, and sometimes unsightly, places. All that is needed is for someone to recognize and acknowledge what others overlook as mundane, or gross, or beneath their curiosity. My teachers were able to do this, and had the devotion, creativity and articulation to convey their appreciation in a way that inspired.

And inspired I was. I desperately wanted to tell these stories that I felt had been passed to me, but I wanted to do it with a visual, fine art approach. For as much as I've focused on anatomy in this narrative, painting is my other great love. I live painting. I breathe painting. From grade school to grad school, from adolescence to adulthood, fine art has been the constant in my life. It's a way for me to express joy when I'm happy, it's a way to find solace when I'm down. My husband knows that if I'm in a funk, the fastest way out of it is to just put a paintbrush in my hand.

So when, in the space of five months, I finished grad school, married, moved across the country, got pregnant, and found out there were severe problems with my pregnancy, it was unsurprising that I turned to painting to restore myself. My first child was born early, weighing just two pounds and five ounces, and spent 72 days in the hospital. At this point, I had taken a break from fine art for a few years, for my graduate program focused on animation and web development, which was generally agreed to be the future of medical illustration. But when despair crept into my heart during those long days and nights in the NICU, I turned to art as an outlet. I wanted to focus on the progress my son was making, on those two steps forward, rather than the one step back. Painting what was going well in his body, rather than focusing on problem areas, allowed me to do this. I started making fine art anatomy—and a decade later, have not yet stopped.

Eventually I decided to share those paintings with the masses, and was able to capture an attentive audience. I created Lyon Road Art, my business that distributes my prints and paintings around the world, named after the street I lived on when my son was in the hospital. I now have a studio space in Waunakee, Wisconsin where I teach and paint with a team of three women. I'm lucky that I'm now able to live my passion by highlighting the beauty of anatomy through traditional painting methods, encouraging in my audience a love for the small dramas happening inside ourselves, a thousand times a day.

Some stories, however, were still beating a drum within me, for I can't always convey the intricacies of physiology through color and form as thoroughly as I want. For me, poetry was the natural next step. Just the multisyllabic names of some structures inspired me with their musical rhythm. (Cusp of Carabelli, anyone?) The more I ruminated on them, the more these poems began to write themselves. I would be driving, or drying my hair or cooking dinner and little stanzas would unfurl in my mind and I'd repeat them feverishly to myself so as not to forget the lines before I could reach my computer. I worked to find crevices in my days between painting and parenting and business-running where I could write. Three years later, I've managed to compile these 100 poems with accompanying paintings that showcase how, in both form and function, anatomy is beautiful.

So in addition to artist, instructor and business owner, I now tentatively add poet to my list of professions. I'd like to think, though, that these occupations can all fall under one umbrella: that of storyteller. I find that as I get older, I simply yearn to be a teacher in the style of those that most motivated me. A narrator of the commonplace turned fascinating, a chronicler of the secret world teeming with life that had just been hiding behind a banal screen. I want to take the torch that I've been lucky enough to recognize and hang on to, the torch of understanding and inspiration and passion, and pass it on to the viewers and readers of my work.

I hope these sometimes silly, sometimes thoughtful, always informative poems inspire you to love and appreciate if not anatomy, then at least the inner machinations of things that are often overlooked.

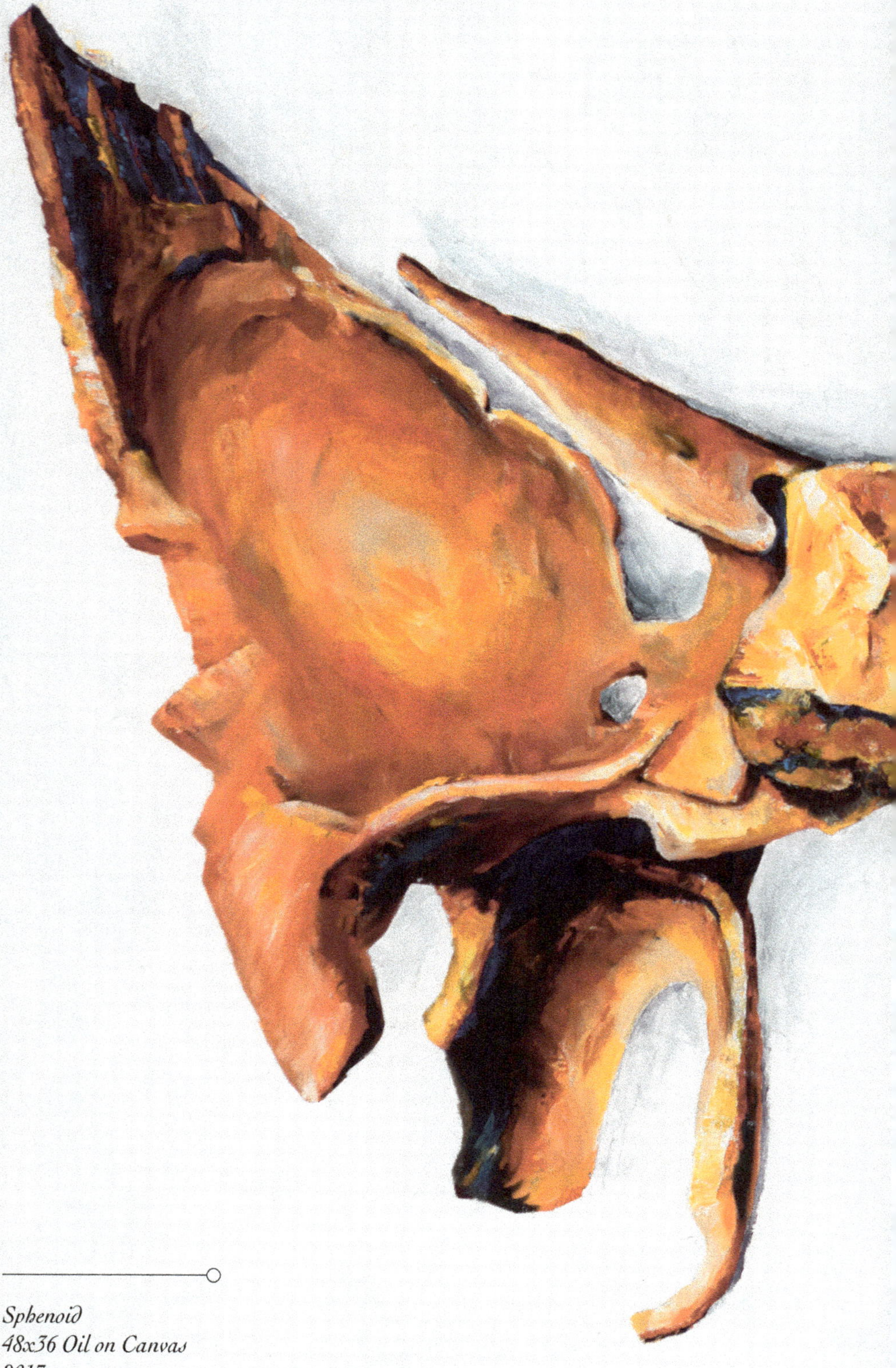

Sphenoid
48x36 Oil on Canvas
2017

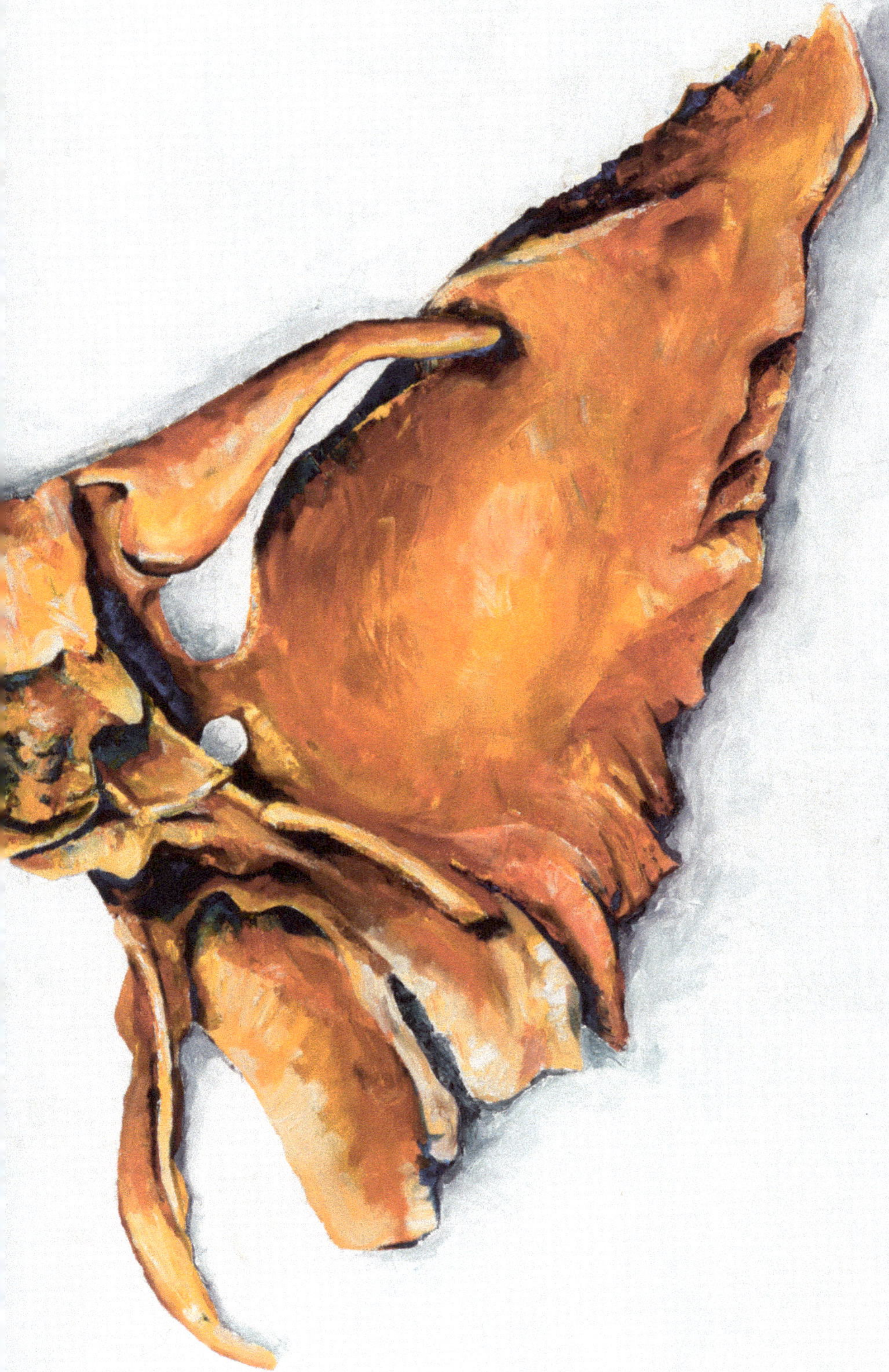

TABLE OF CONTENTS

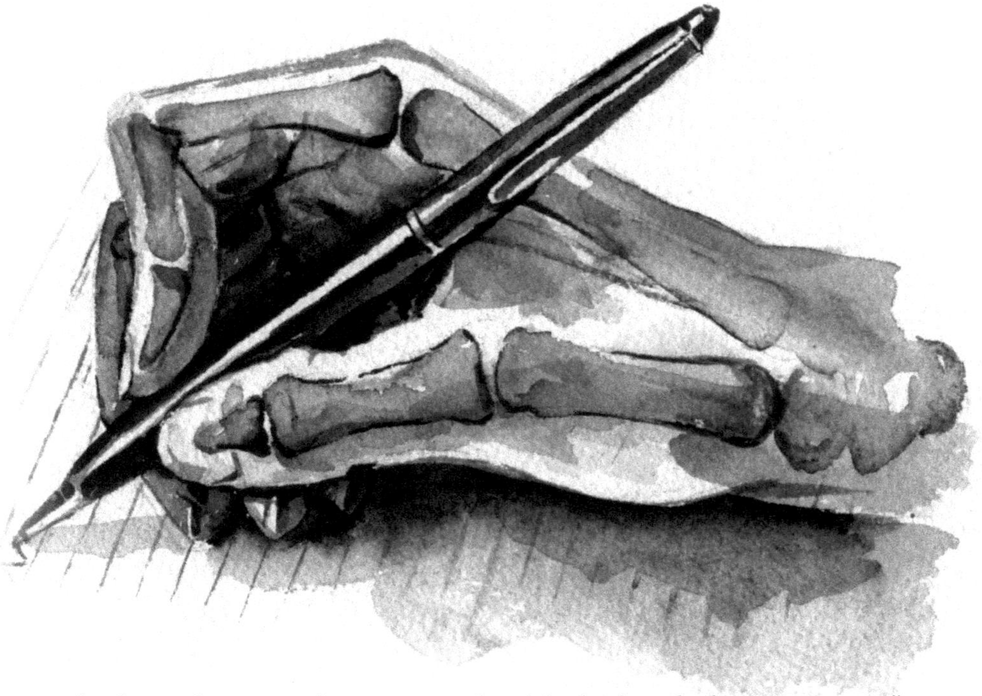

"Where the spirit does not work with the hand, there is no art."
-Leonardo Da Vinci

Writing Hand
7x5 Watercolor
2021

ANATOMY IS BEAUTIFUL

Anatomy is more
than a framework.
It tells a story
of our similarities
and our singularity.
It is organized
but chaotic;
it is profound,
yet overlooked.
But most of all,
for those who care to see,
anatomy
is
beautiful.

Cervical Spine
5x10 Watercolor
2021

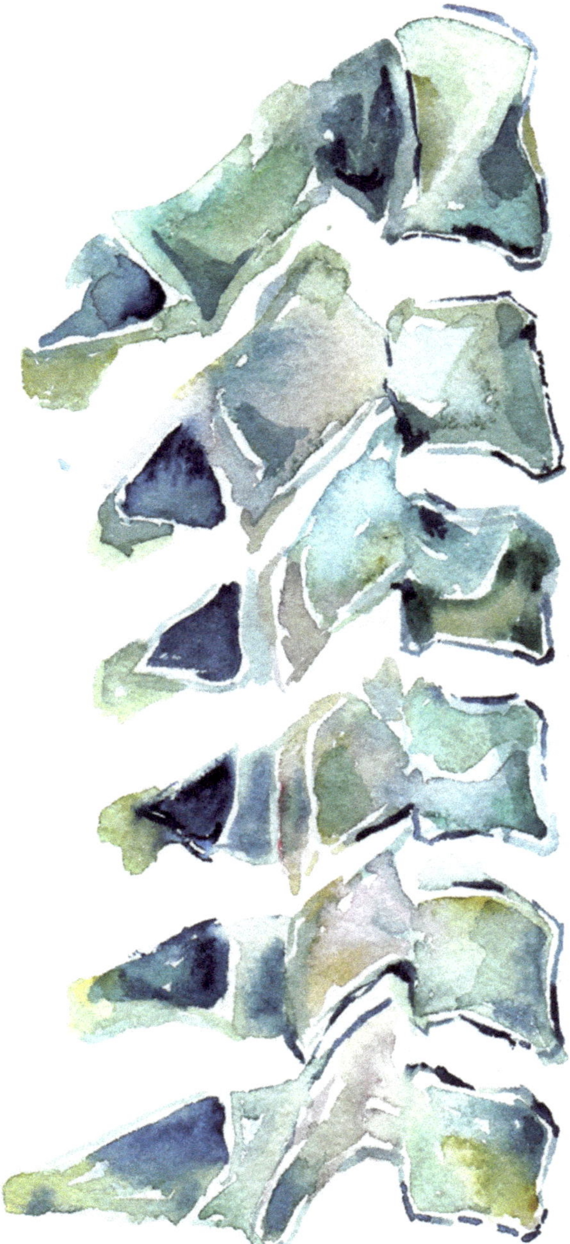

chapter one

MUSCLES & TENDONS

"I have been impressed with the urgency of doing. Knowing is not enough, we must apply. Being willing is not enough, we must do."

-Leonardo Da Vinci

MUSCLES WITH WEIRD NAMES PART I

Platysma is abysmal
At making a face look happy.

Anconeus gets acrimonious
Because his elbow job is crappy.

Obturator is the operator
Of keeping the femur in place.

Multifidus is meticulous
About being the spine's best brace.

Popliteus admits he does
A lot to stabilize the knee.

Pectineus is pretty, plus
She's a crucial leg adductee.

Sternocleidomastoid has a factoid:
He's the strongest neck muscle by far.

Gastrocnemius is dreamiest,
The lower leg's biggest star.

Buccinator's the creator
Of blowing, sucking motions

Risorius is notorious
For giving the mouth some emotion.

Saying muscle names are fun.
But for now I think I'm done.

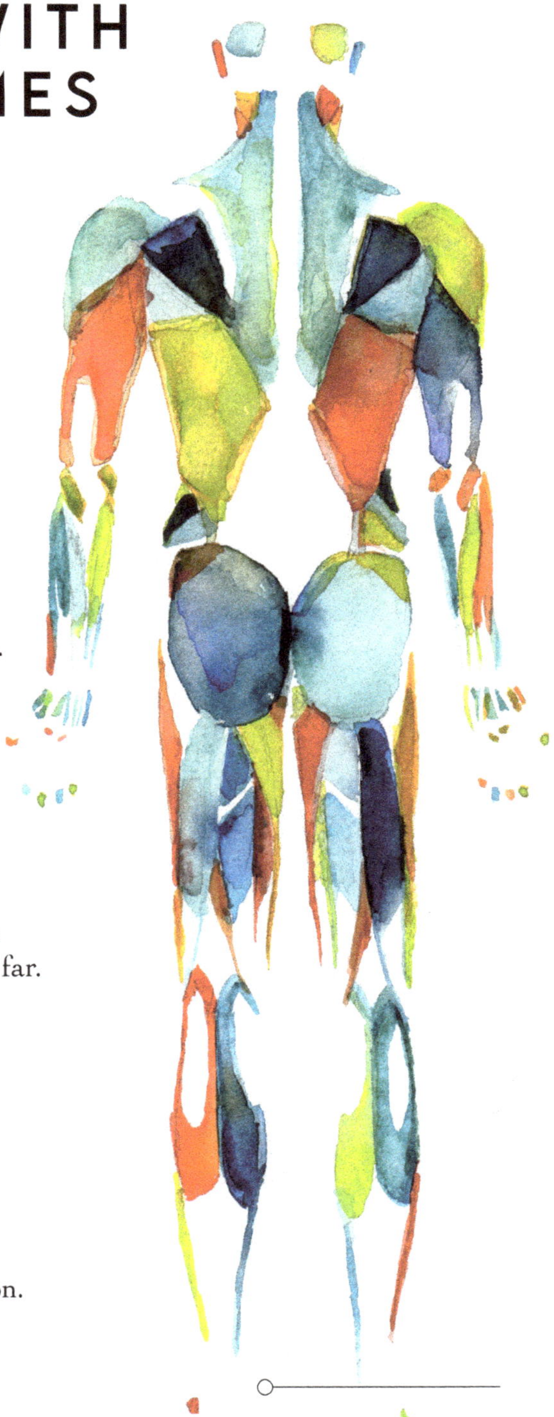

Muscles in Red, Blue and Green
8x10 Watercolor
2018

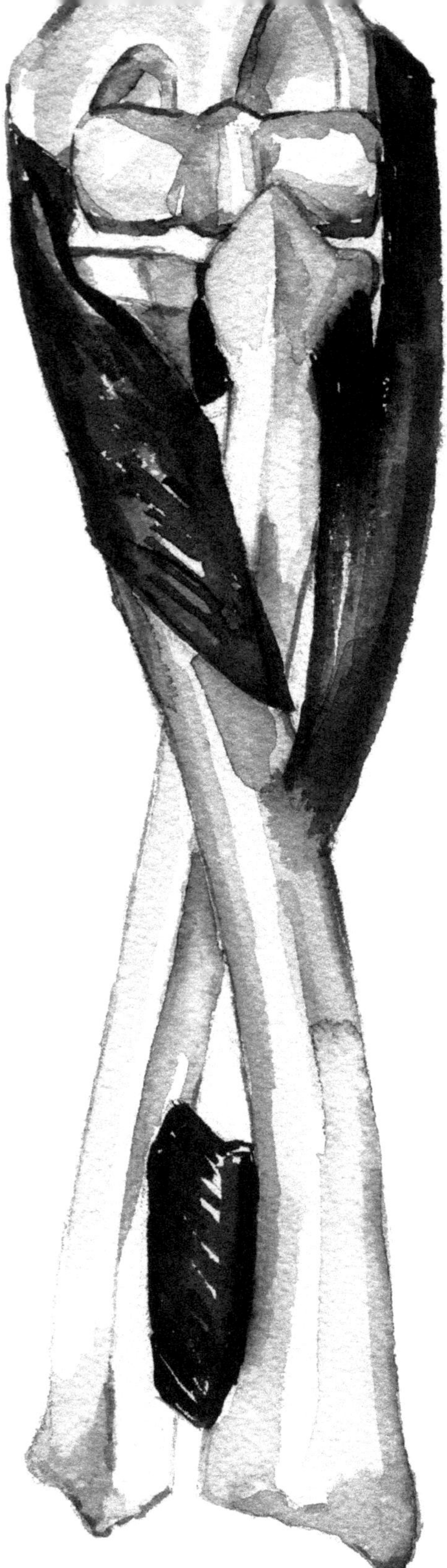

THE TWIST

My hand turns up,
My hand turns down.
A twist that's unique
To the forearm.

To make the palm
Turn to the sky,
The supinator
Is the guy.

To make the palm
Spin to the floor,
Two muscle friends
Are up to the chore.

First of the pair:
Pronator Quadratus.
He's the strongest
And the fattest.

But he needs support
From his buddy,
Pronator Teres,
Long and ruddy.

When these three muscles
Work as a team
The radius can twirl
At the ulnar seam.

The Twisters
8x10 Watercolor
2018

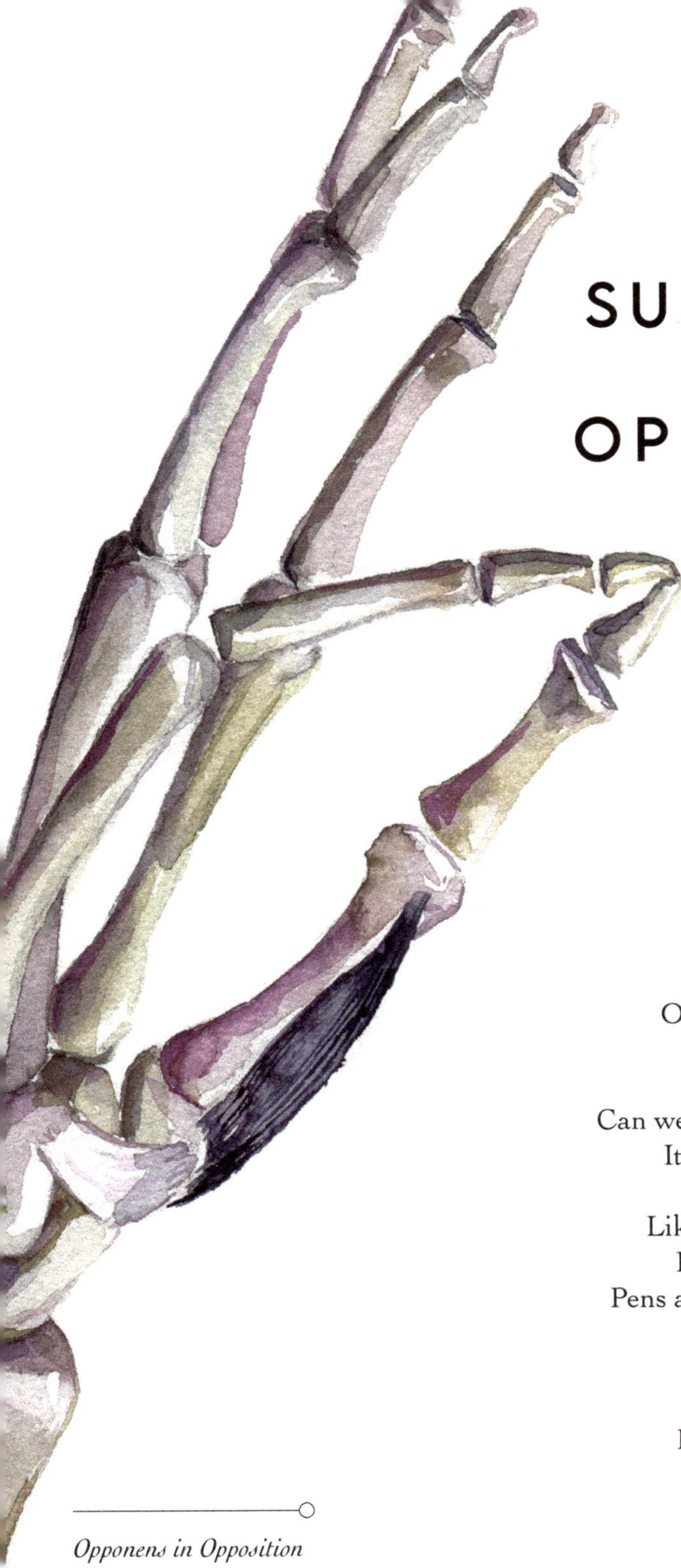

SUPPOSIN' ON THE OPPONENS

I was just supposin'...
What if Opponens
Didn't do its job?

If it doesn't contract,
The thumb can't contact
The nearby finger-tops.

That pincer position,
Named opposition,
Is all Opponens' doin'.

And each time it flexes
It adds to the nexus
Of what makes us human.

For only with a grasp
Can we hold, squeeze and clasp
Items that make life swell.

Like guitars and good beer,
Hands that we hold dear,
Pens and paintbrushes as well.

So I was supposin'
Without the opponens
Life would be rather sad.

Opponens in Opposition
6x10.5 Watercolor
2023

CONVERSATION WITH A PT

You need to strengthen your pelvic floor.
But I already work out—must I do more?
Well, do you leak when you jump, sneeze or laugh?
Wait, pelvic floor strength will help with that?
Yes, and better sex too, I have to mention.
All right, you have my attention.
And I assume you don't want a pelvic prolapse?
You'll have to remind me—pray, what is that?
Some organs fall into your vagina and stay.
Um, okay, I'll do whatever you say!
Great! First, pretend that you're peeing.
You're weird. But if it helps my wellbeing…
Now try and stop it mid-stream.
Oh! When I clench, I see what you mean!
That move strengthens the levator ani.
I'm assuming that is the main guy?
Yes, also there's coccygeus too.
Whatever. Is that all I have to do?
Yup, just do ten kegels three times a day.
That sounds exhausting. Is there another way?
Well, I could stimulate it with electrodes in your rectum.
You know what? Kegels sound fun!

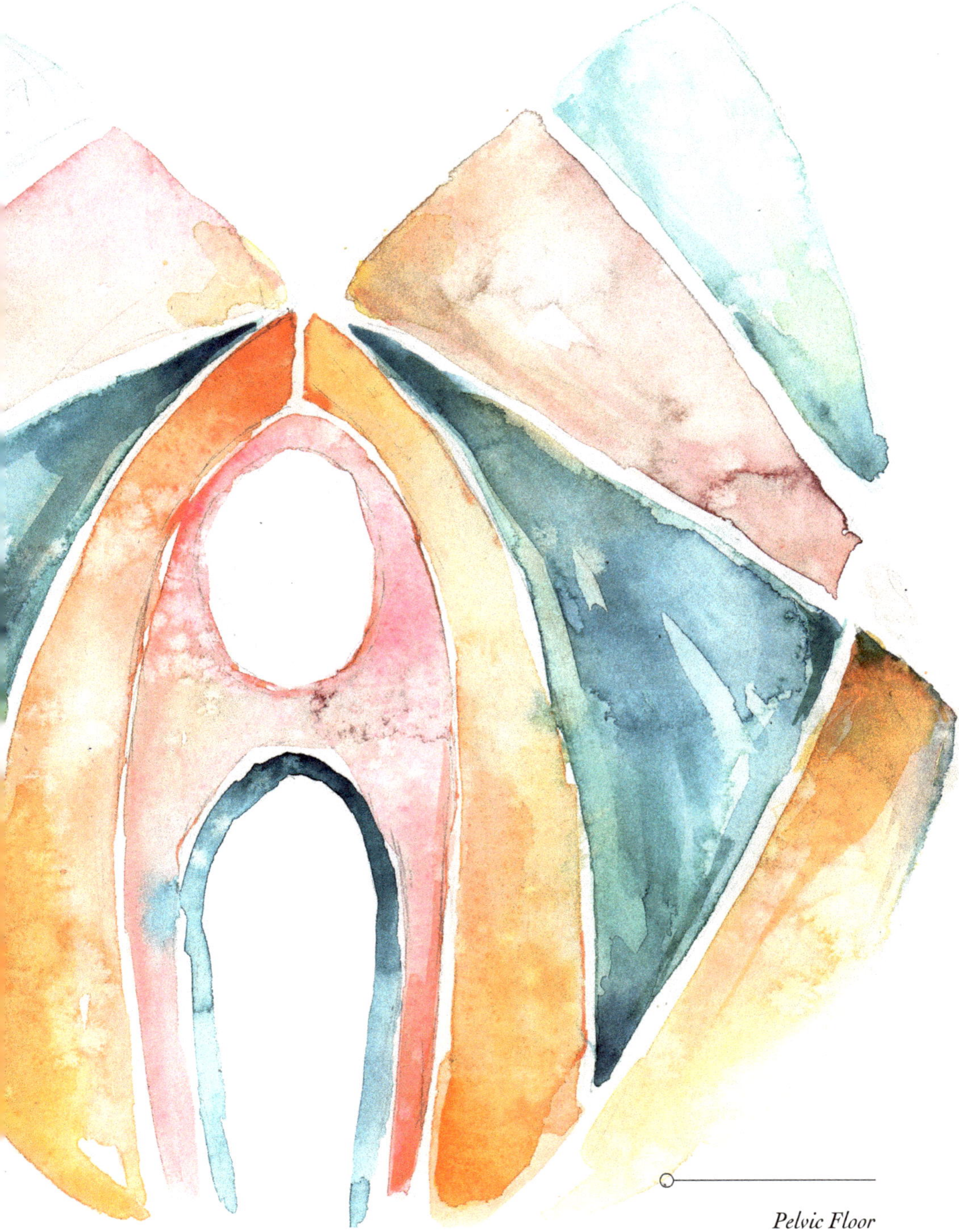

Pelvic Floor
10x10 Watercolor
2019

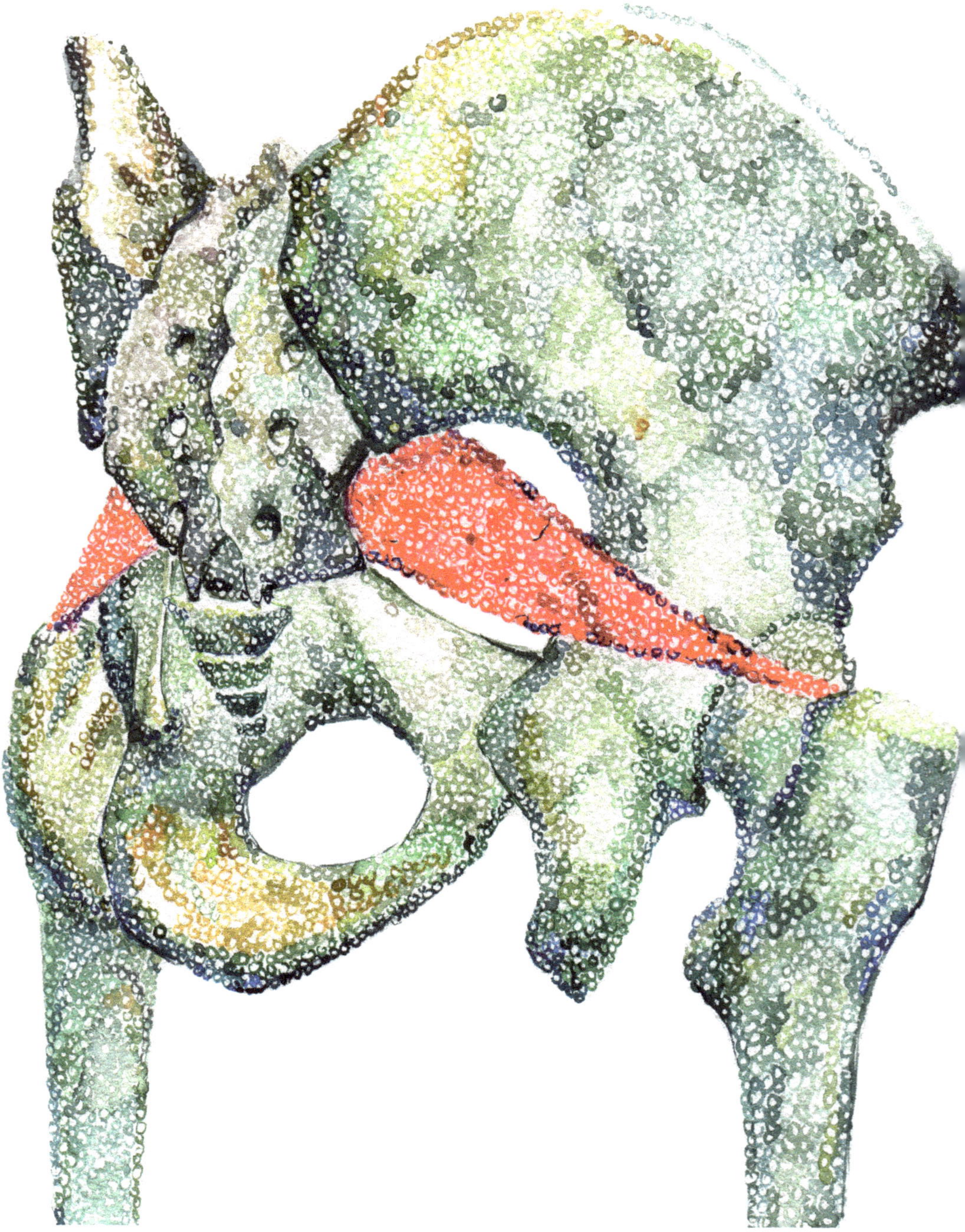

Piriformis
8x10 Watercolor
2024

PIRIFORMIS

For Dawn. Sorry about your piriformis.

The piriformis
Is not enormous.
It's not imposing,
And far from foreboding.
It may be a tragedy,
But it just lacks the majesty
Of the gluteal boors
That live next door.
Sure, the leg it twists
But you get the gist—
It's just not the champ
Of the buttocks camp.
But though the muscle's not
Quite the cream of the crop,
Imagine you slipped...
And the piriformis ripped...
After you fell...
IT WOULD HURT LIKE HELL.

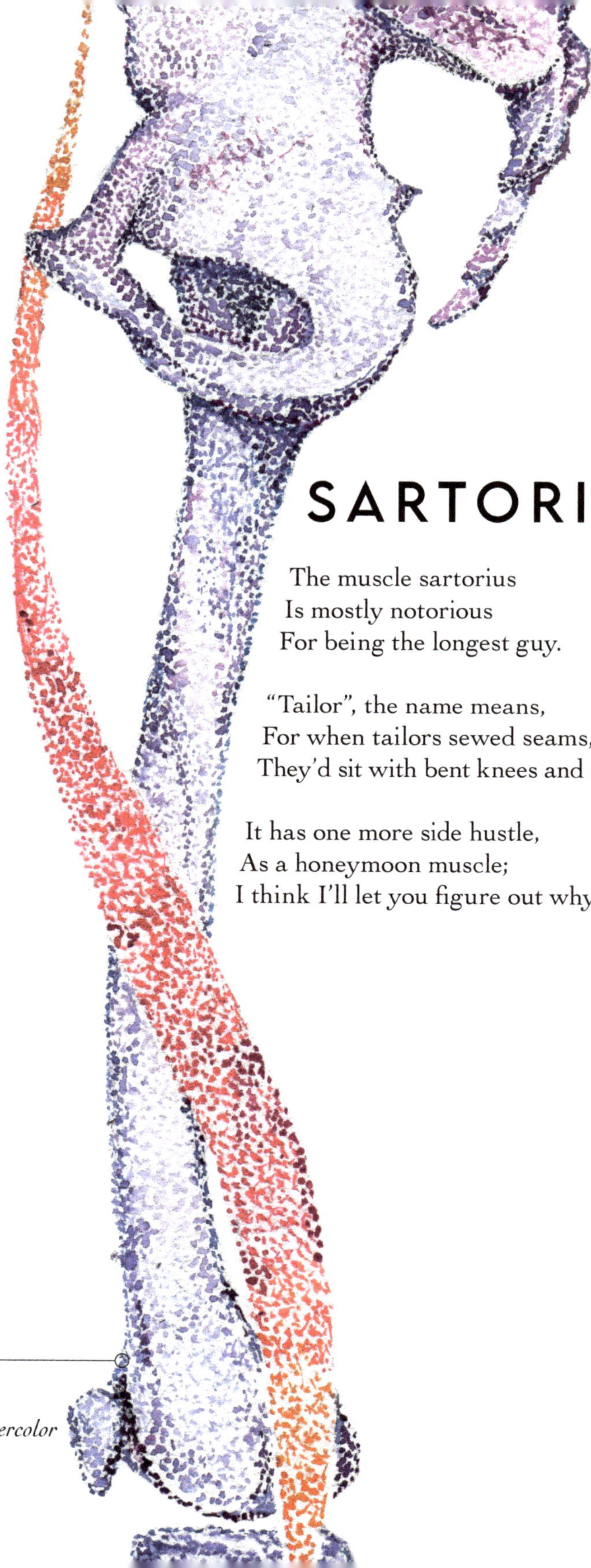

SARTORIUS

The muscle sartorius
Is mostly notorious
For being the longest guy.

"Tailor", the name means,
For when tailors sewed seams,
They'd sit with bent knees and spread thighs

It has one more side hustle,
As a honeymoon muscle;
I think I'll let you figure out why.

Sartorius
8x10 Watercolor
2024

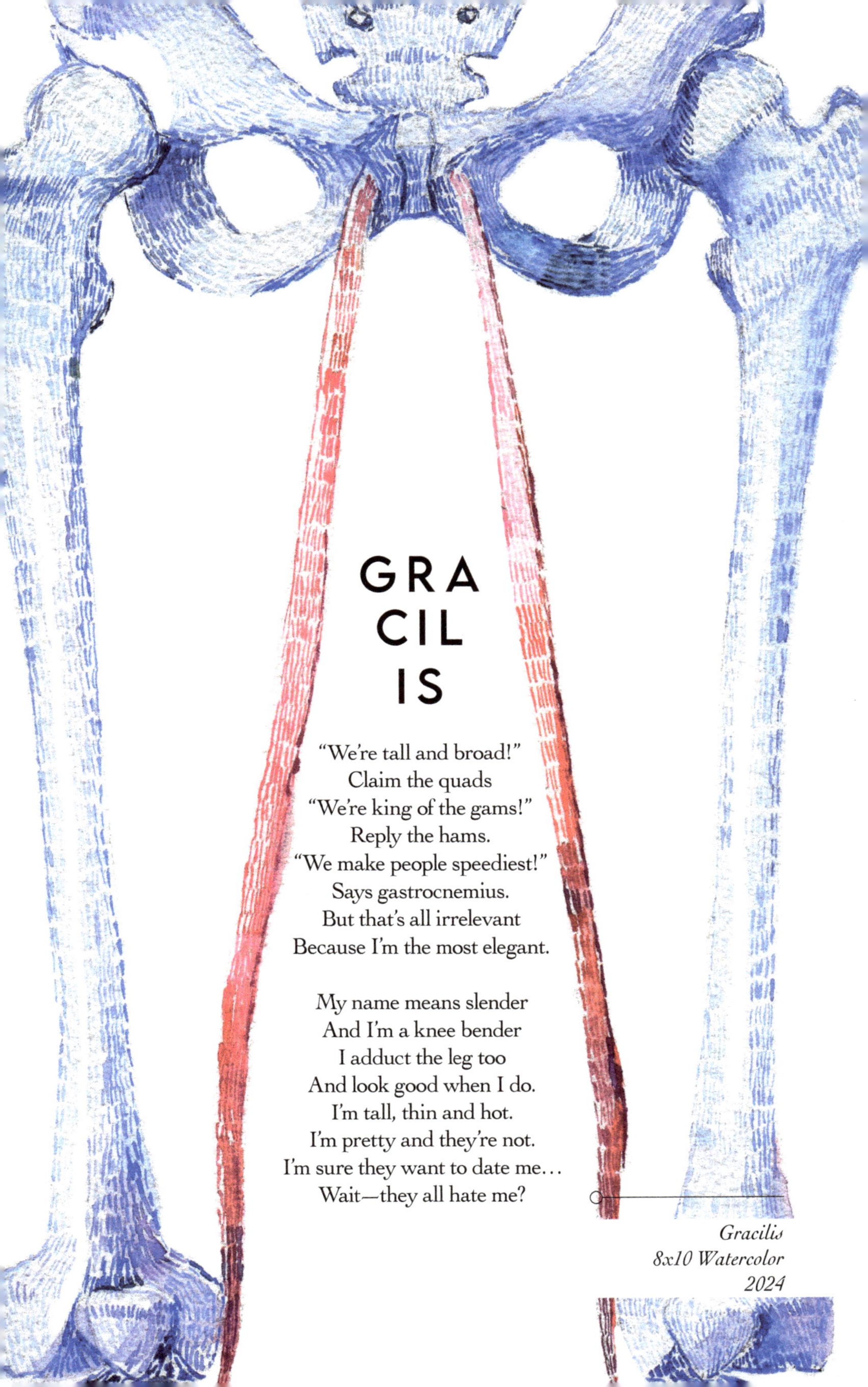

GRA CIL IS

"We're tall and broad!"
Claim the quads
"We're king of the gams!"
Reply the hams.
"We make people speediest!"
Says gastrocnemius.
But that's all irrelevant
Because I'm the most elegant.

My name means slender
And I'm a knee bender
I adduct the leg too
And look good when I do.
I'm tall, thin and hot.
I'm pretty and they're not.
I'm sure they want to date me…
Wait—they all hate me?

Gracilis
8x10 Watercolor
2024

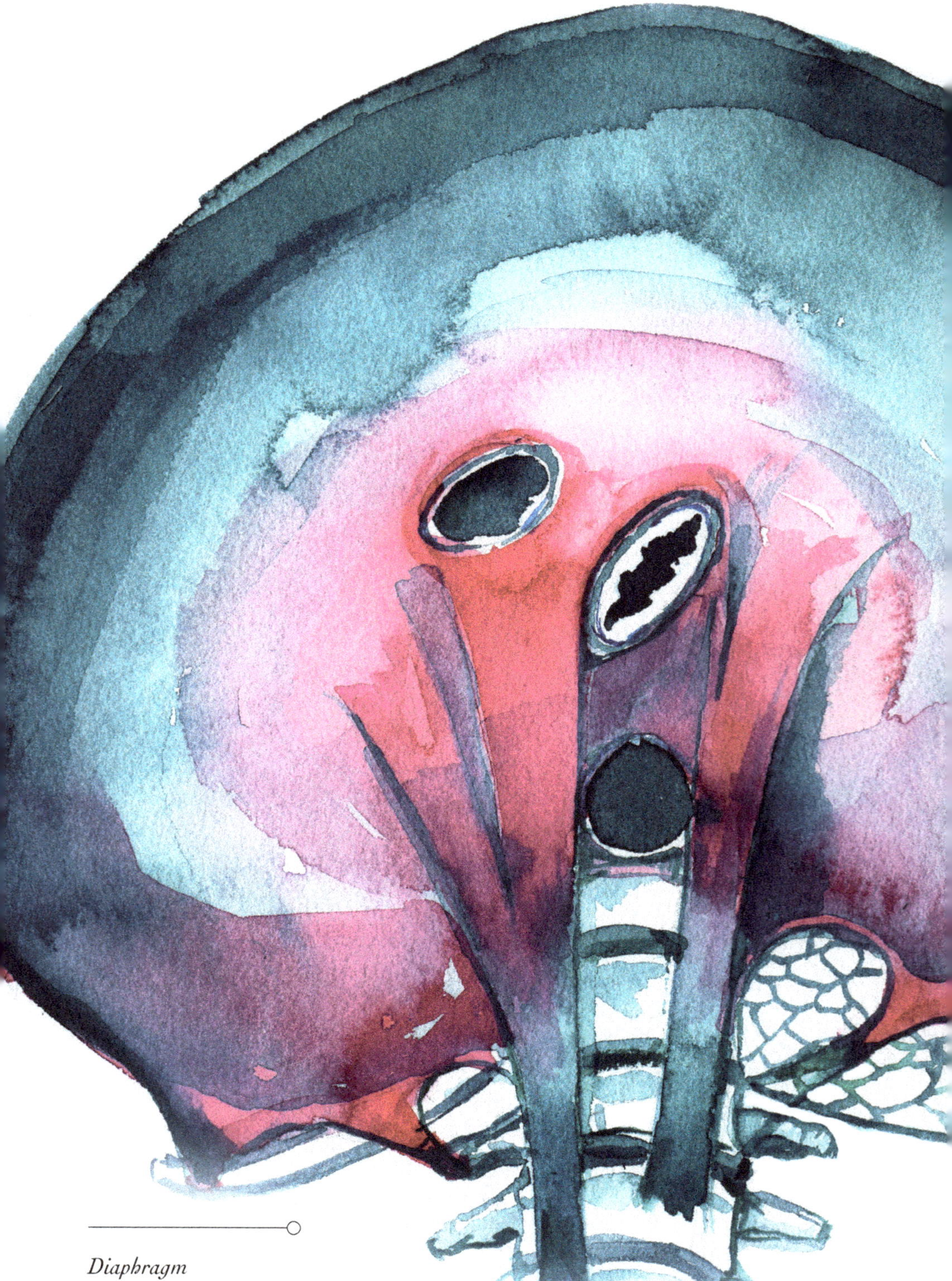

Diaphragm
10x8 Watercolor
2024

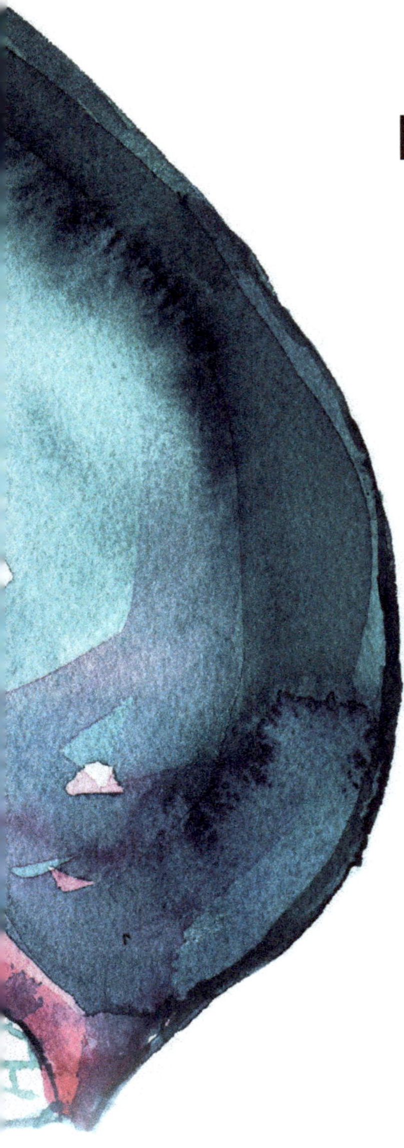

DIAPHRAGM

She lifts,
Lungs expand.
She drifts,
And they land.

She's a muscle
Of great renown
As she hustles
Up and down.

When air is near
But feels short,
When it's fear
That you court,

A strong pull
Of her sheet
Will null
Panic's heat.

Breathing
Is magic
When your heaving's
Diaphragmatic.

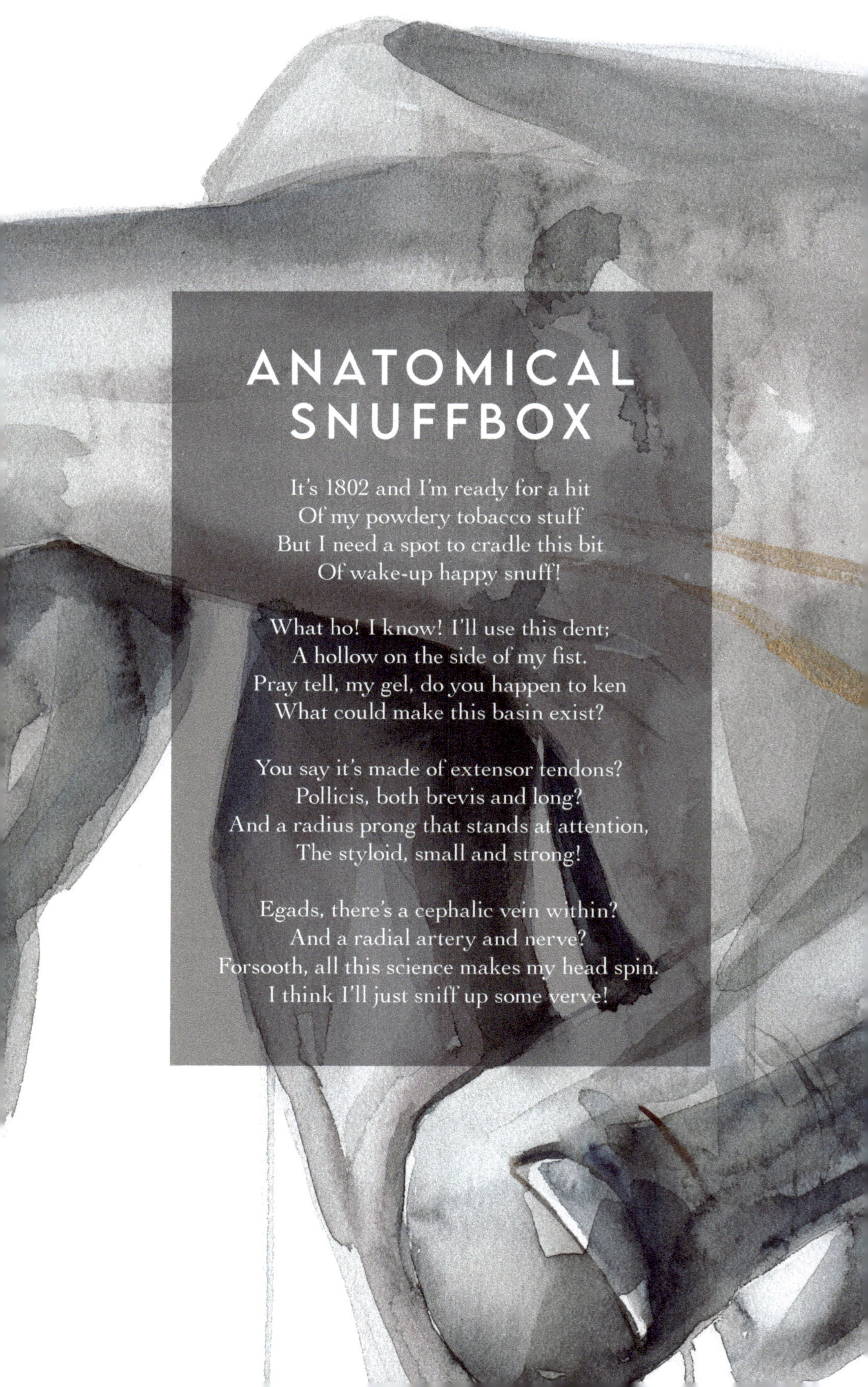

ANATOMICAL SNUFFBOX

It's 1802 and I'm ready for a hit
Of my powdery tobacco stuff
But I need a spot to cradle this bit
Of wake-up happy snuff!

What ho! I know! I'll use this dent;
A hollow on the side of my fist.
Pray tell, my gel, do you happen to ken
What could make this basin exist?

You say it's made of extensor tendons?
Pollicis, both brevis and long?
And a radius prong that stands at attention,
The styloid, small and strong!

Egads, there's a cephalic vein within?
And a radial artery and nerve?
Forsooth, all this science makes my head spin.
I think I'll just sniff up some verve!

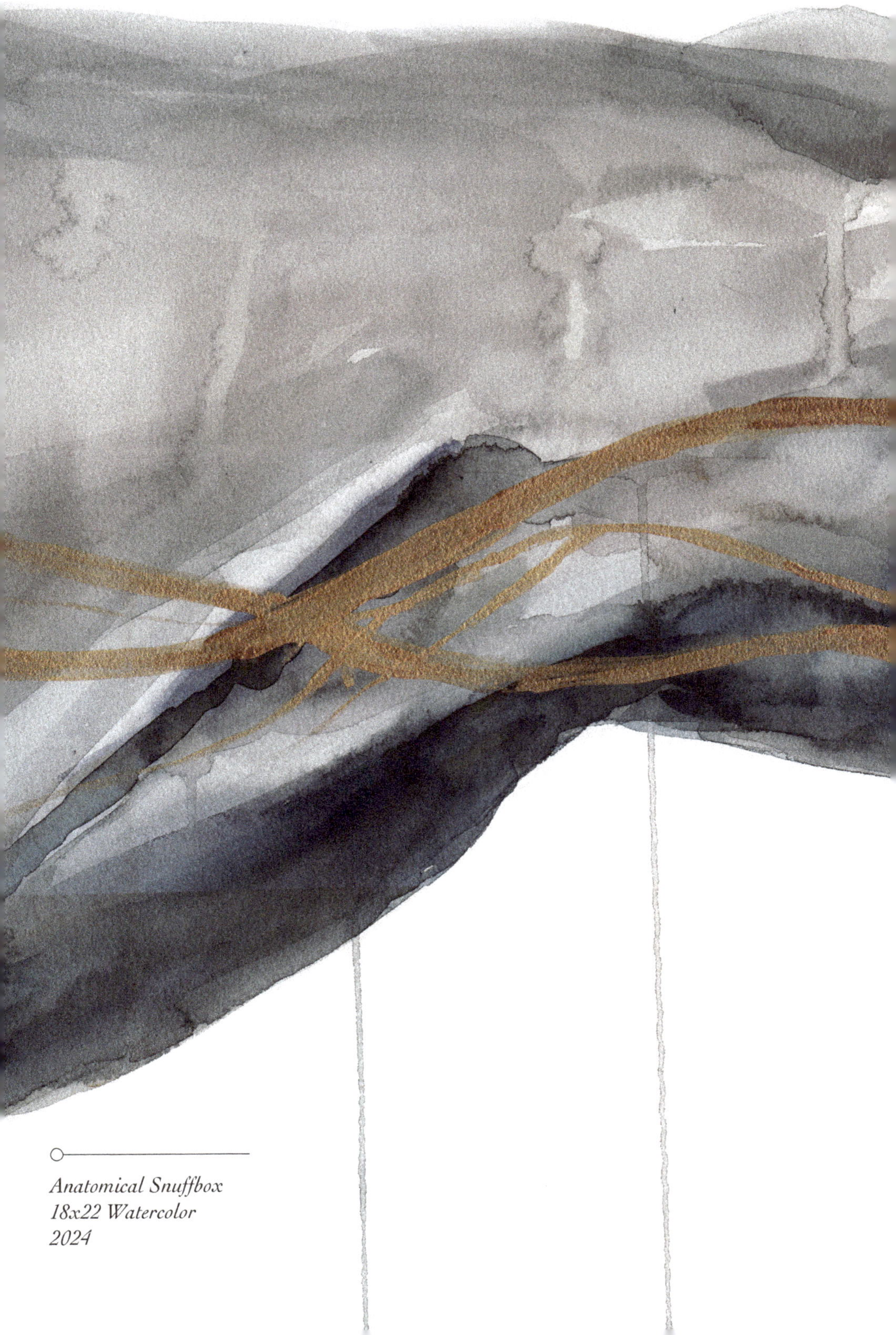

Anatomical Snuffbox
18x22 Watercolor
2024

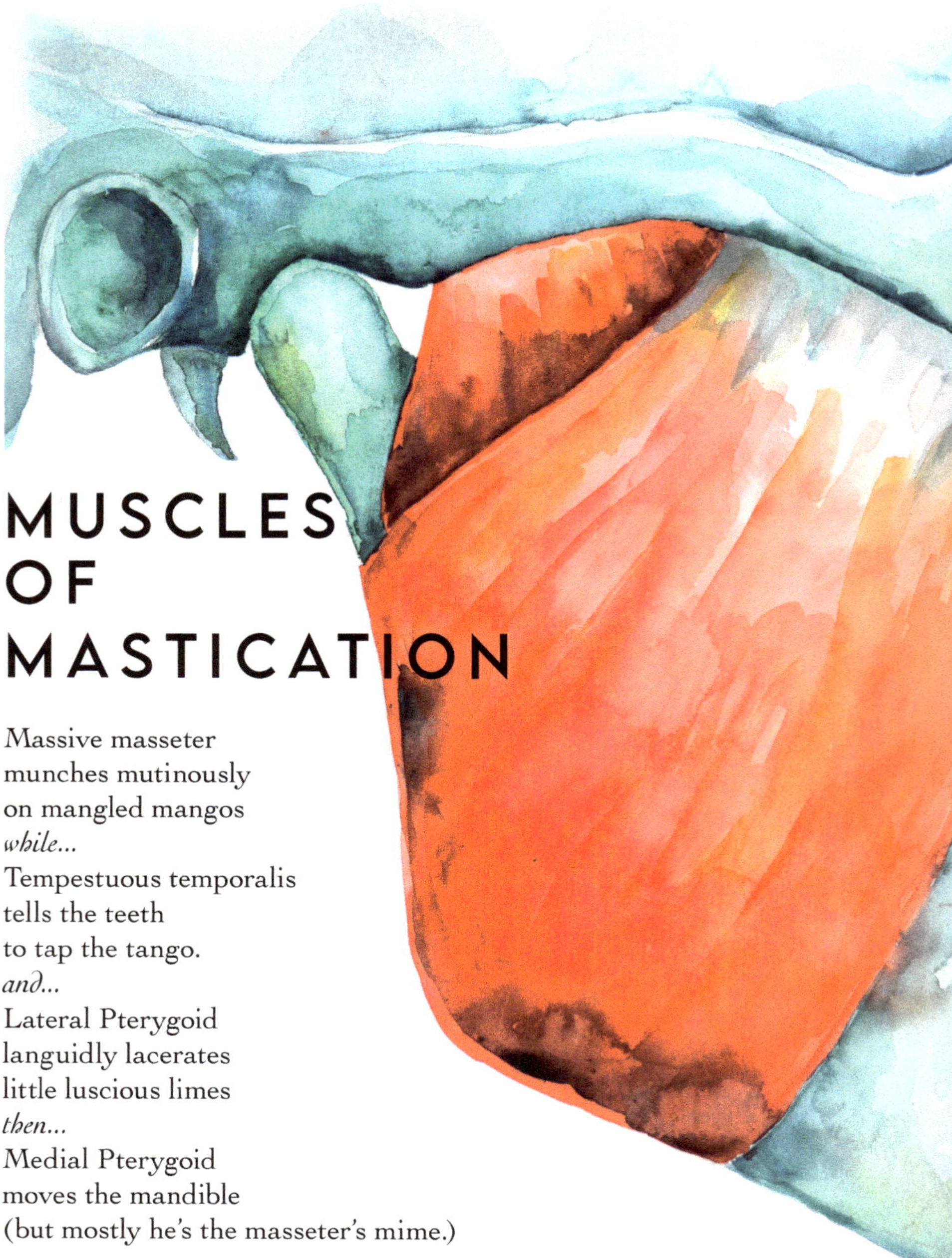

MUSCLES OF MASTICATION

Massive masseter
munches mutinously
on mangled mangos
while...
Tempestuous temporalis
tells the teeth
to tap the tango.
and...
Lateral Pterygoid
languidly lacerates
little luscious limes
then...
Medial Pterygoid
moves the mandible
(but mostly he's the masseter's mime.)

Masseter
22x30 Watercolor
2016

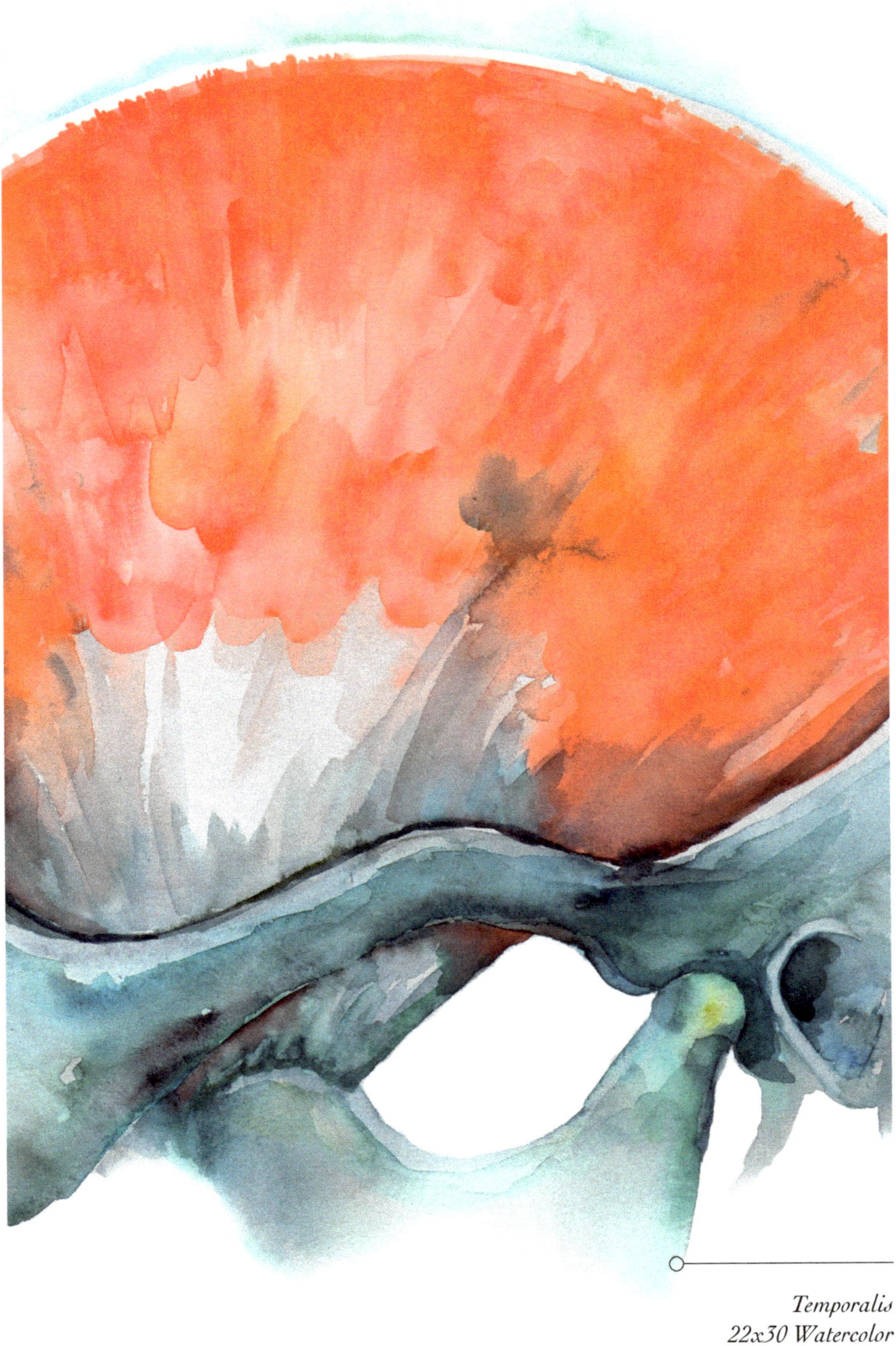

Temporalis
22x30 Watercolor
2016

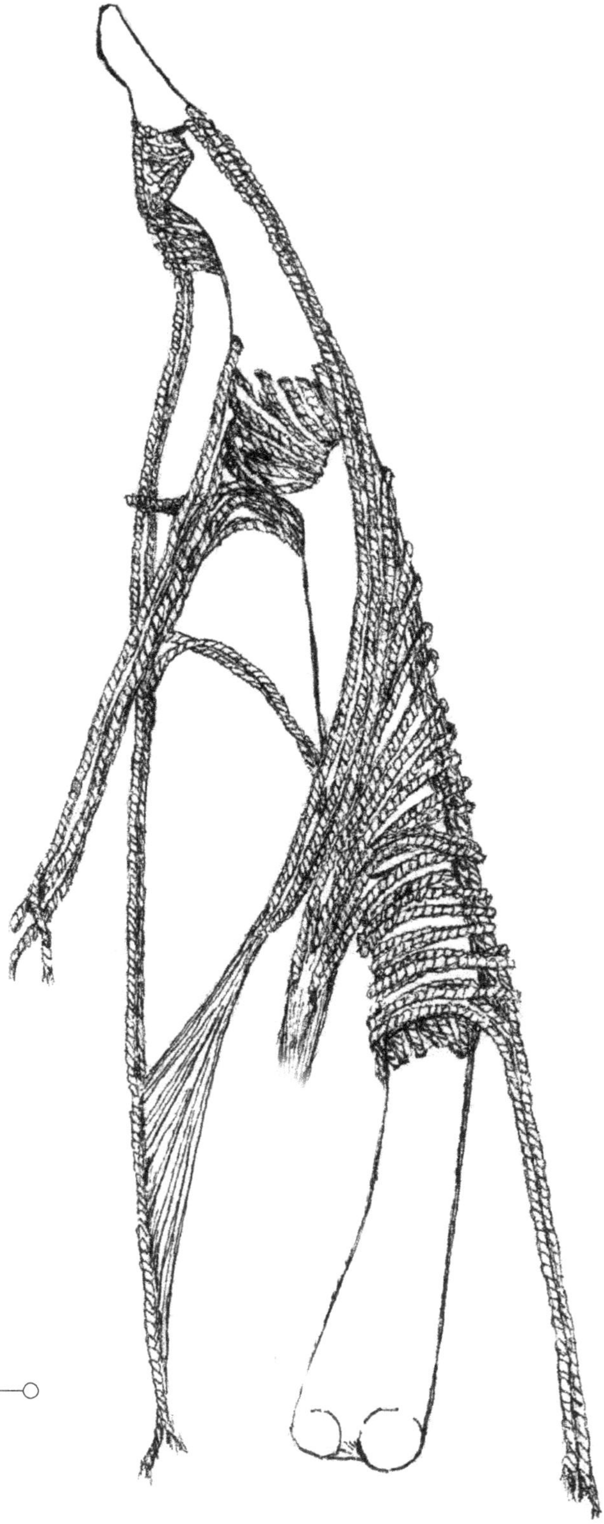

Lumbrical Ropes
8x10 Pen & Ink
2024

HEAVE! HO!

We lumbricals toil and sweat
        In the belly of the Palmar Hand
We extend, yes, but also flex
        The finger joints, on command.

Heave! Ho! We push! We pull!

With a heave we force an intrepid bend
        Of digits at the MP joint.
With a ho the IP joints extend,
        Ensuring a finger can easily point.

Heave! Ho! We push! We pull!

Our long, white, tendonous oars
        Allow these paradoxical motions
For they traverse the MP ridge's floor
        Then ascend the extensor expansion.

Heave! Ho! We push! We pull!

Our tendons continue their stalwart climb,
        Almost reaching the dorsal plane.
But at last plunge into the finger's side,
        To join the lateral band's extension train.

Heave! Ho! We push! We pull!

Thus our long, perilous knuckle crossing,
        And our endurance and lack of temerity,
Yield opposing motions without pausing,
        And add to the hand's dexterity.

Heave! Ho! We push! We pull!

LONG NAME

There's a lot of muscles on which I'm hazy
But there's one I know 'cause its name is crazy.
It dilates the nose so you can smell daisies.
Though it is small, its title is weighty.
By the end of saying it my eyes get glazy.
I'd write it out but I'm tired and lazy.
Ok, fine…
Levator labii superioris alaeque nasi.

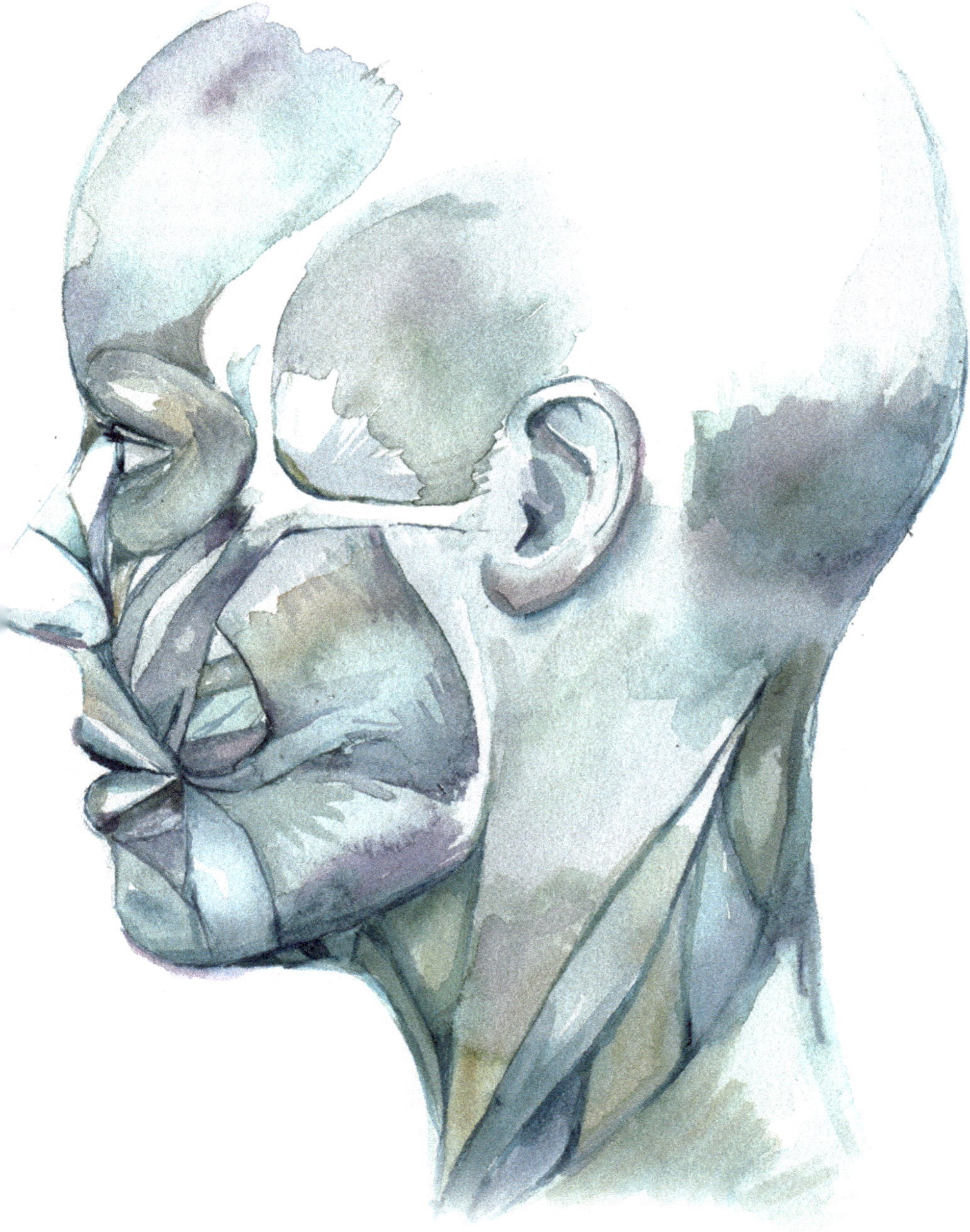

Profile of the Facial Muscles
11x14 Watercolor
2024

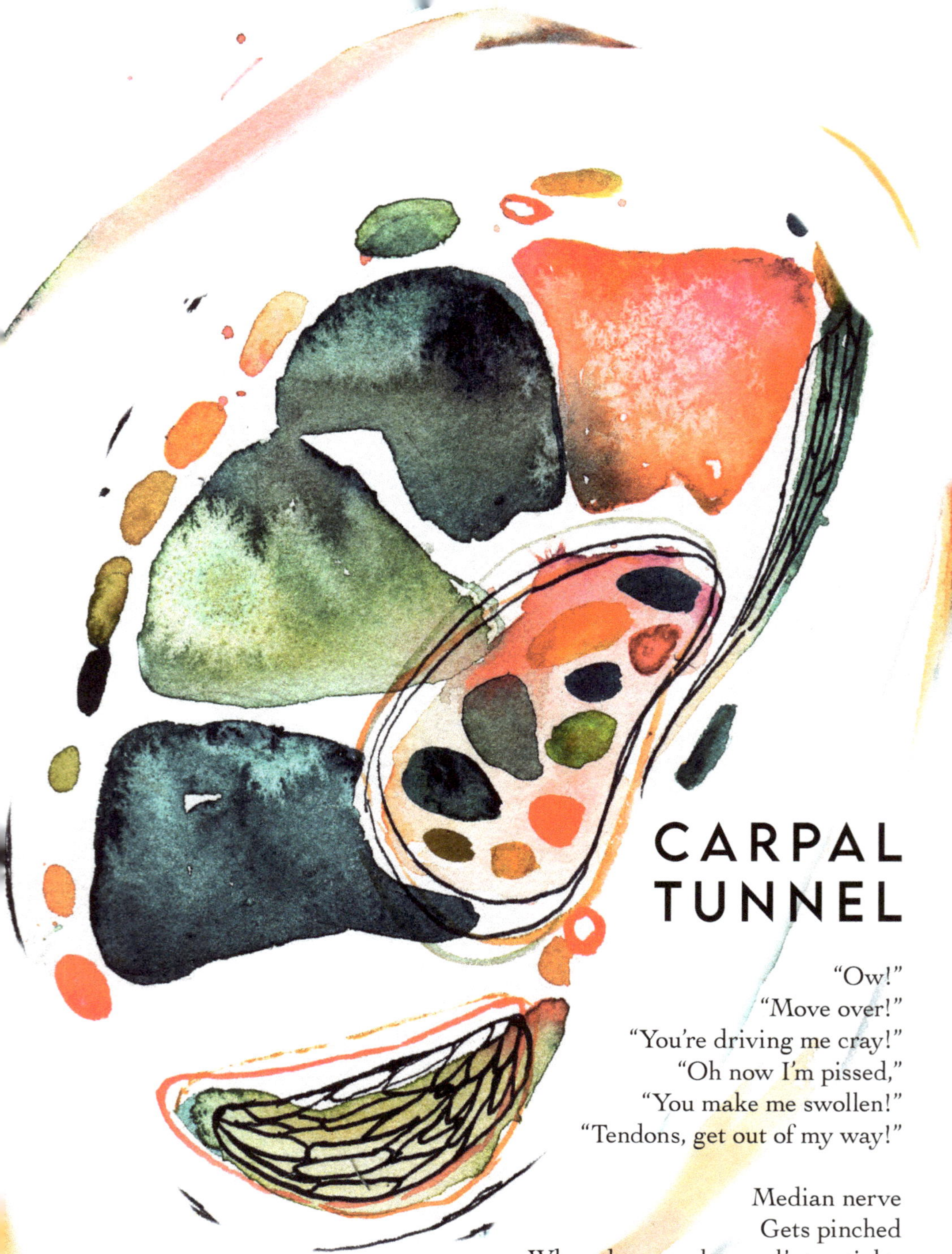

CARPAL TUNNEL

"Ow!"
"Move over!"
"You're driving me cray!"
"Oh now I'm pissed,"
"You make me swollen!"
"Tendons, get out of my way!"

Median nerve
Gets pinched
When the carpal tunnel's too tight.
Whoever decided
to design it like this…
I really would like to fight.

Cross Section of the Wrist
8x10 Watercolor
2024

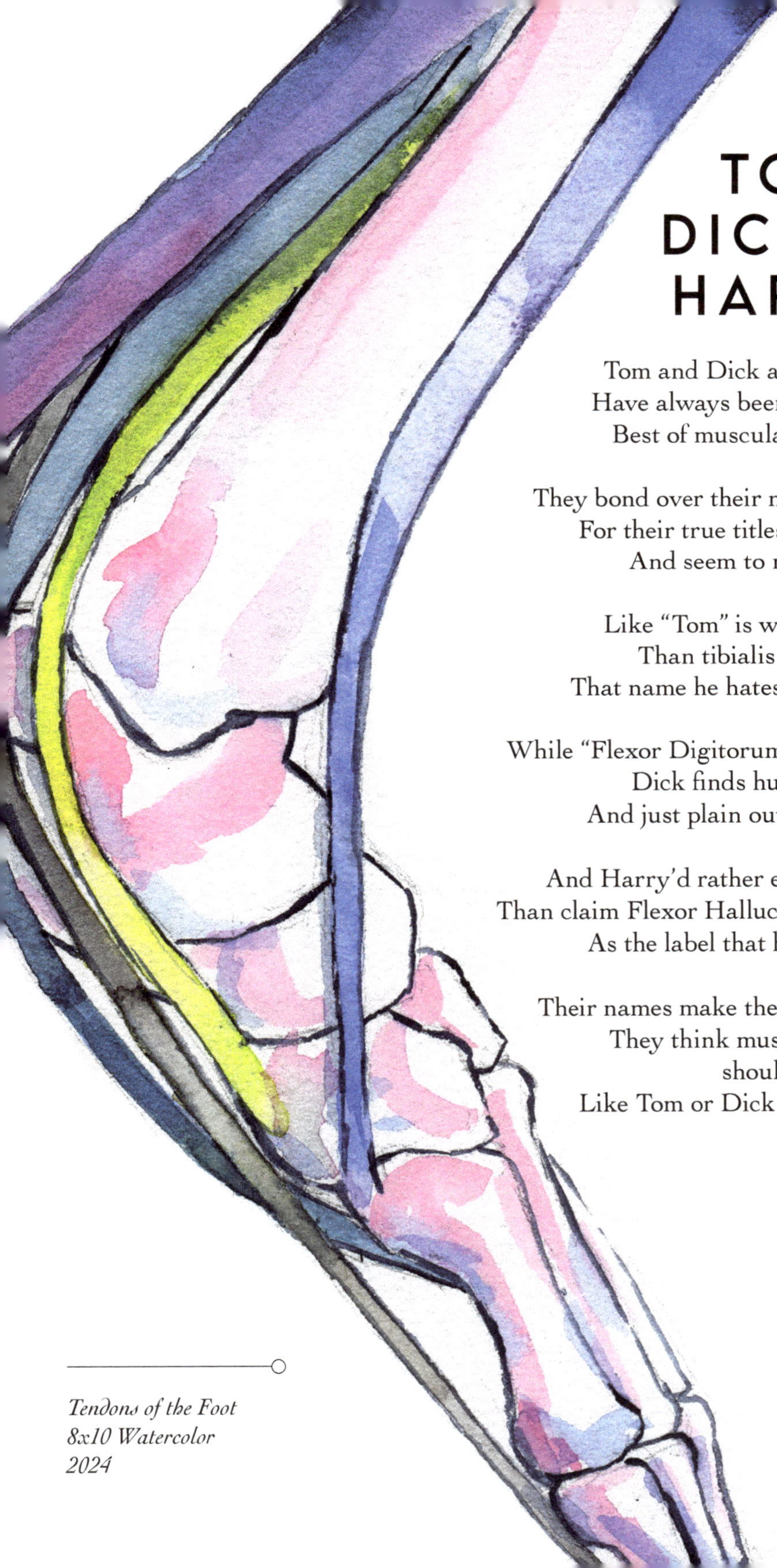

TOM, DICK & HARRY

Tom and Dick and Harry
Have always been the very
Best of muscular friends.

They bond over their nicknames
For their true titles are lame
And seem to never end.

Like "Tom" is way clearer
Than tibialis posterior,
That name he hates so much.

While "Flexor Digitorum Longus"
Dick finds humongous,
And just plain out of touch.

And Harry'd rather eat fungus
Than claim Flexor Hallucis Longus
As the label that he carries.

Their names make them queasy.
They think muscle names
should be easy,
Like Tom or Dick or Harry.

Tendons of the Foot
8x10 Watercolor
2024

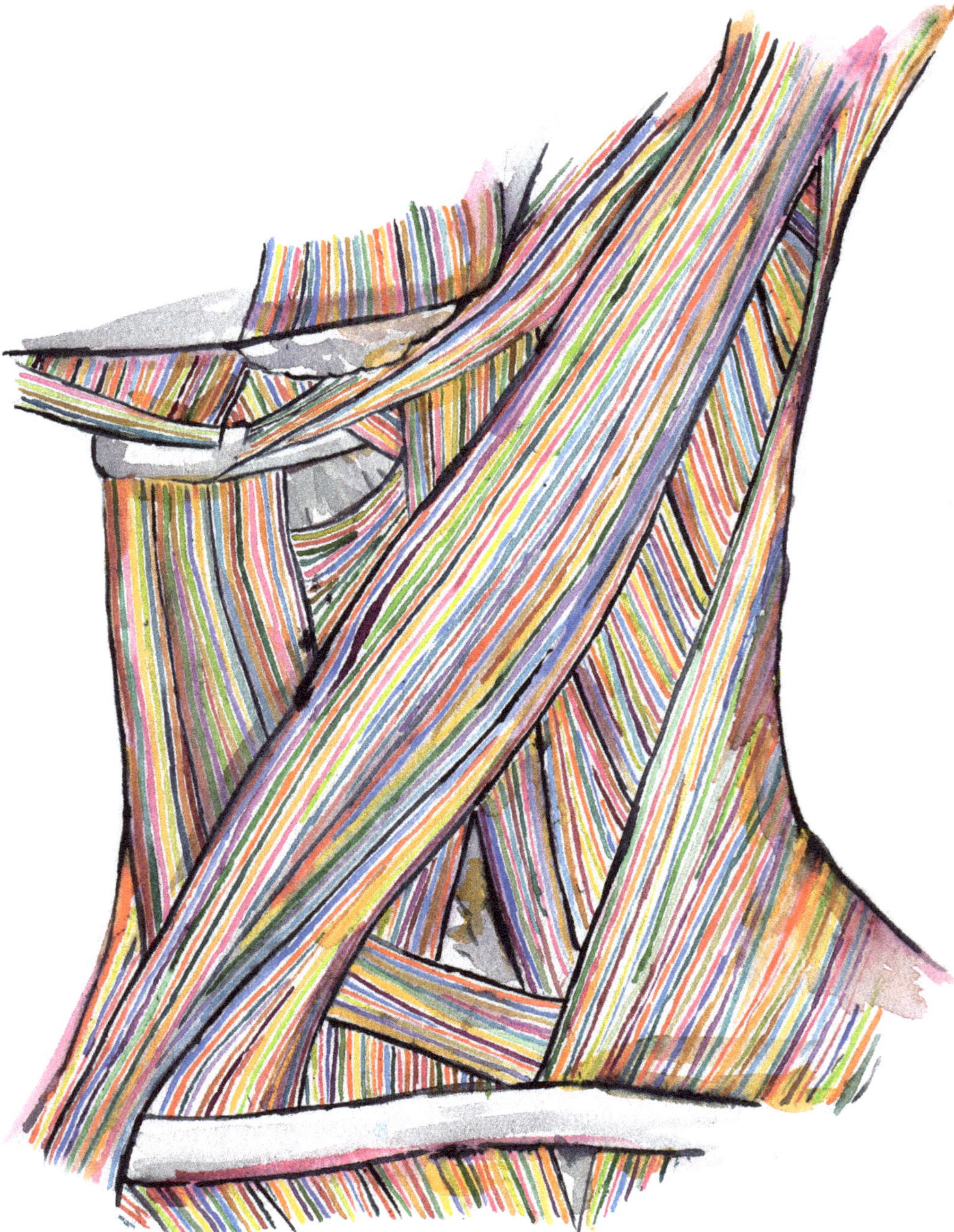

Neck Muscles
11x14 Watercolor
2024

DEAR STERNOCLEIDOMASTOID,

Dear Sternocleidomastoid,
You are stronger than an asteroid
Tough and bold and strong,
You never seem to do wrong.
You rotate the head so boldly,
And flex the neck so nobly.
Yet I feel the urge to cry.
As I watch you from nearby.
For while my love for you persists,
I don't think you know I exist.
And though we share an insertion
I live in fear of your aversion.
So I'll just say it once, very clearly
I admire and love you dearly.
I'll await your final analysis.
Love,
Splenius Capitis

DEAR SPLENIUS CAPITIS,

I've oft been accused of callousness,
So I'll try to be nice, but frank
Thank you, but no thanks.
Sorry if your heart is destroyed.
Best,
Sternocleidomastoid

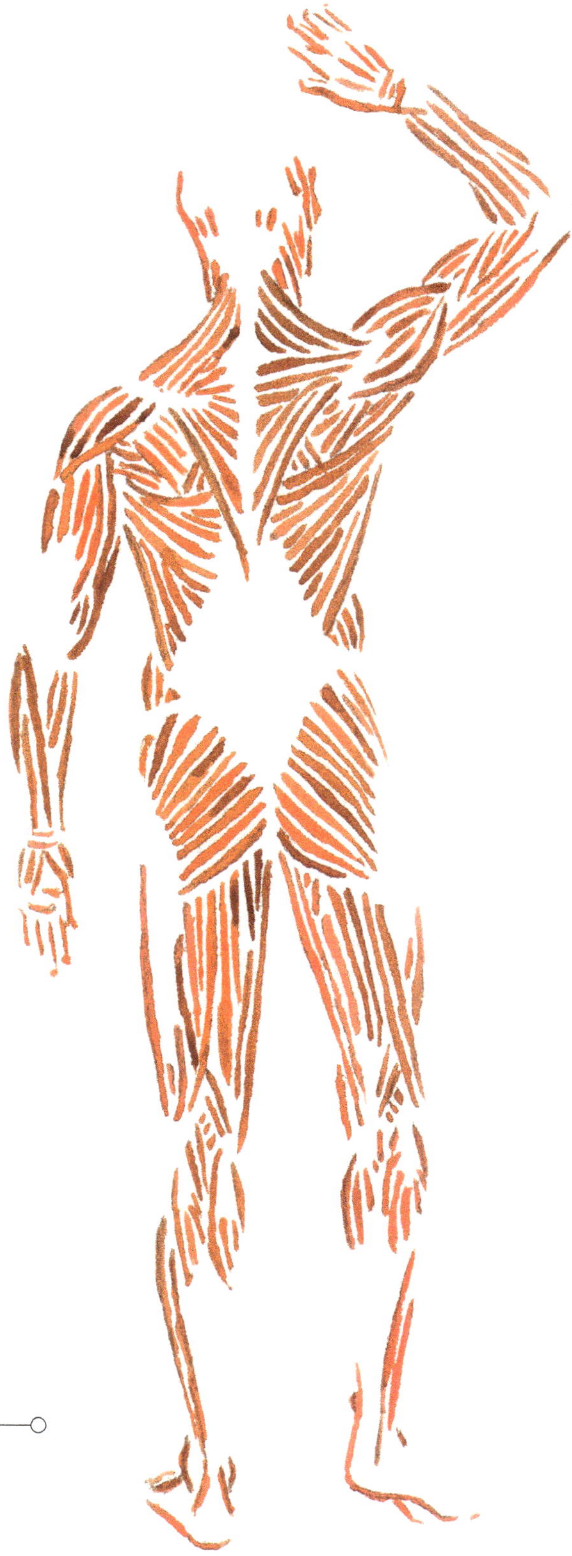

Muscle M
8x10 Wa
2016

MUSCLES WITH WEIRD NAMES PART II

Orbicularis oculi gets a high
From squeezing closed the eyes.

Stapedius is the neediest
For he's the smallest in size.

Coccygues is fastidious
About flexing the coccyx tail.

Pyramidalis has some malice,
As the abdomen's most frail.

The intercostals are hostile
As they force air out of the lungs

Genioglossus is the crossest
As she boldly sticks out the tongue.

Opponens likes supposin'
That he makes the thumb so special.

And levator ani is the guy
Who makes the pelvic floor a vessel.

Intertransversarii hide in the spine,
In the transverse process nooks.

Flexor digitorum profundus has an abundance
Of tendons, to finger crook.

These muscle names twist my tongue.
I think now I'm really done.

chapter two

CELLS & SMALL THINGS

"To develop a complete mind: Study the science of art; Study the art of science. Learn how to see. Realize that everything connects to everything else."

-Leonardo Da Vinci

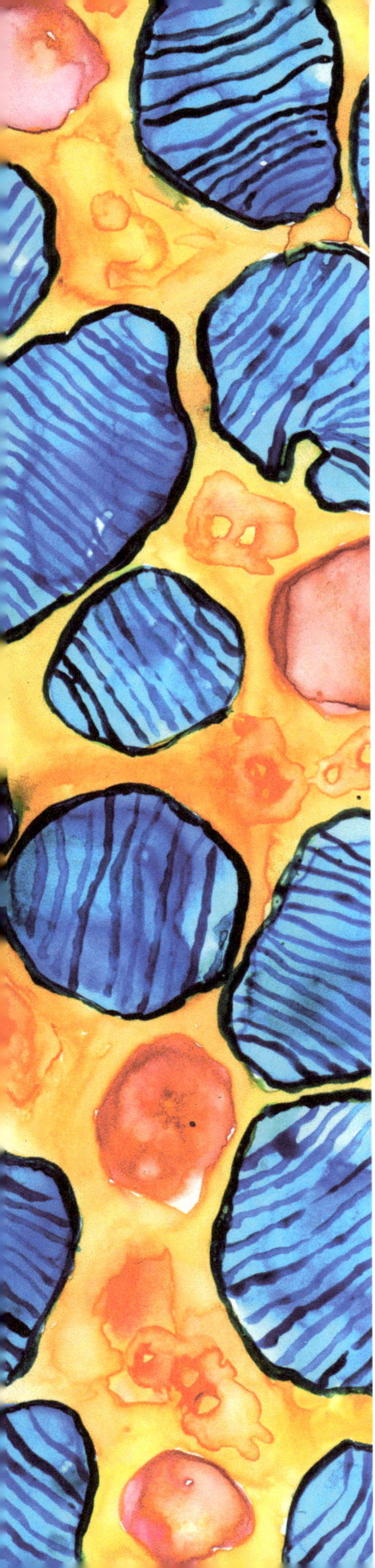

MIGHTY MITOCHONDRION

I'm lively and energetic:
An organelle that's full of fun.
I am rowdy and frenetic,
Me, the mighty mitochondrion.

The harbinger of energy,
Without me food would be just food.
But with some inner synergy,
I take it and make it something good.

In fact, I think I should get a prize
For being awesome every single day,
Since before your eyes I oxidize
Acetyl-Coenzyme A.

Yeah, I take that 'zyme for a ride
Along a pathway I call Krebs.
The reactions I get, I'll confide,
Are better than taking happy meds.

By the end that enzyme will alter
Into adenosine triphosphate.
ATP, for short, and it won't falter
At bringing a party to your gate.

Because ATP is power,
An upper that's full of might!
So trust me, without me, you'd glower,
For I bring the zeal, pep and sprite!

Mitochondria
9x12 Watercolor on Yupo
2017

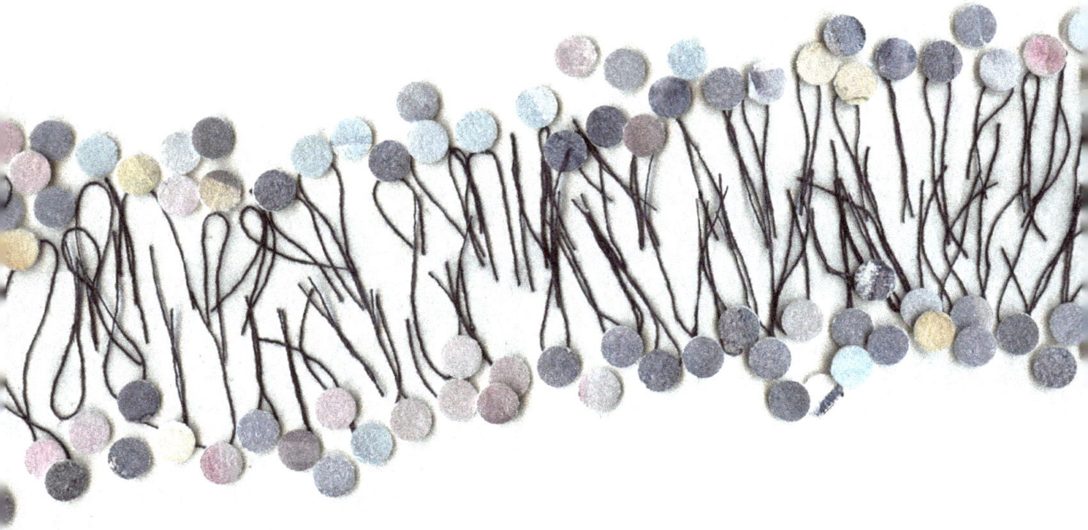

SEMIPERMEABLE PHOSPHOLIPID BILAYER

The cell membrane is like a wall
(But don't call it that—it's not a plant!)
To all organelles inside its fold,
Endless protection it will freely grant.

I recall my teacher called it
"A semipermeable phospholipid bilayer."
That's a mouthful of slippery syllables
So let's break it down to the main players.

Semipermeable means it's snooty
About who gets to get through the fence.
Only small or hydrophobic molecules
Can diffuse past its fatty defense.

A Cell Membrane
13x5 Mixed Media
2024

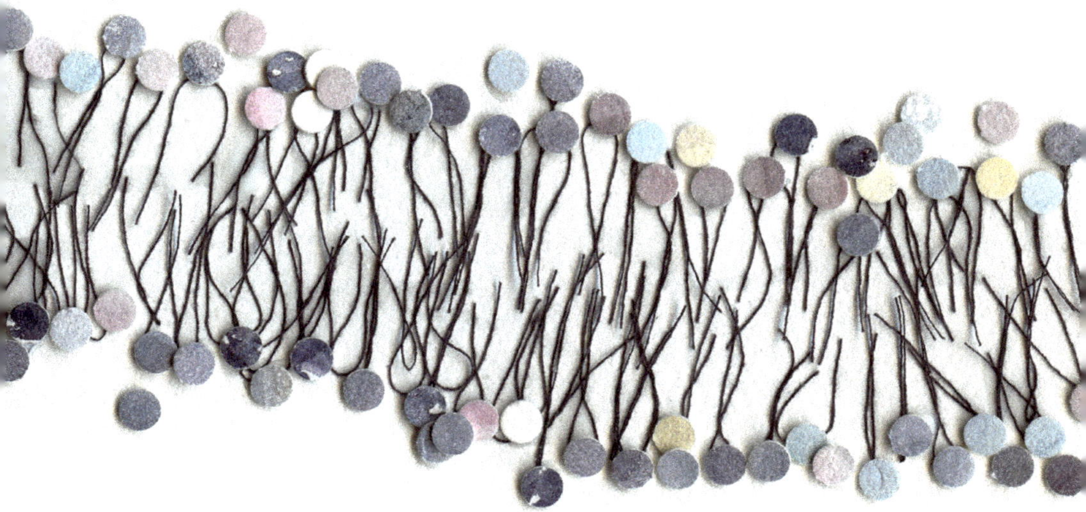

It's all due to wee phospholipids,
Whose two components make it idyllic:
The tails that turn away from water
And the head that's hydrophilic.

The tails all want to snuggle together
Away from the water found inward and out
So the heads face out, forming two rows,
And that's how the bilayer all comes about.

Packed like sardines, they protect the cell,
With the help of proteins stuck in their midst
Spitting out toxins that will only do harm.
And letting the good stuff in for a tryst.

OVERKILL, DUDE

I'm just a mast cell, but please don't mind me.
Just keeping a look out, casual as can be.
Do I have the most important job here?
Hunting down pathogens, KILLERS you fear?
ABSOLUTELY YES, but it's no big deal
I'm just one of the guys— with WEAPONS to wield!
Don't worry, everything's as it should be,
No invaders as far as I can—

WHAT THE $!@*& WAS THAT?????
ENEMY SIGHTED!
RELEASE THE HISTAMINE! GO GO GO!
SPRAY IT EVERYWHERE, I DON'T CARE!!!
JUST GET EM! KILL THEM
BEFORE THEY KILL US!!!

Oh... wait... was that just another peanut?
And now you're swollen, itchy, can't breathe? But...
You're alive at least! Now, don't give me attitude
Ok fine. Yeah, I know. Overkill, dude.

Degranulating Mast Cells
16x20 Watercolor
2016

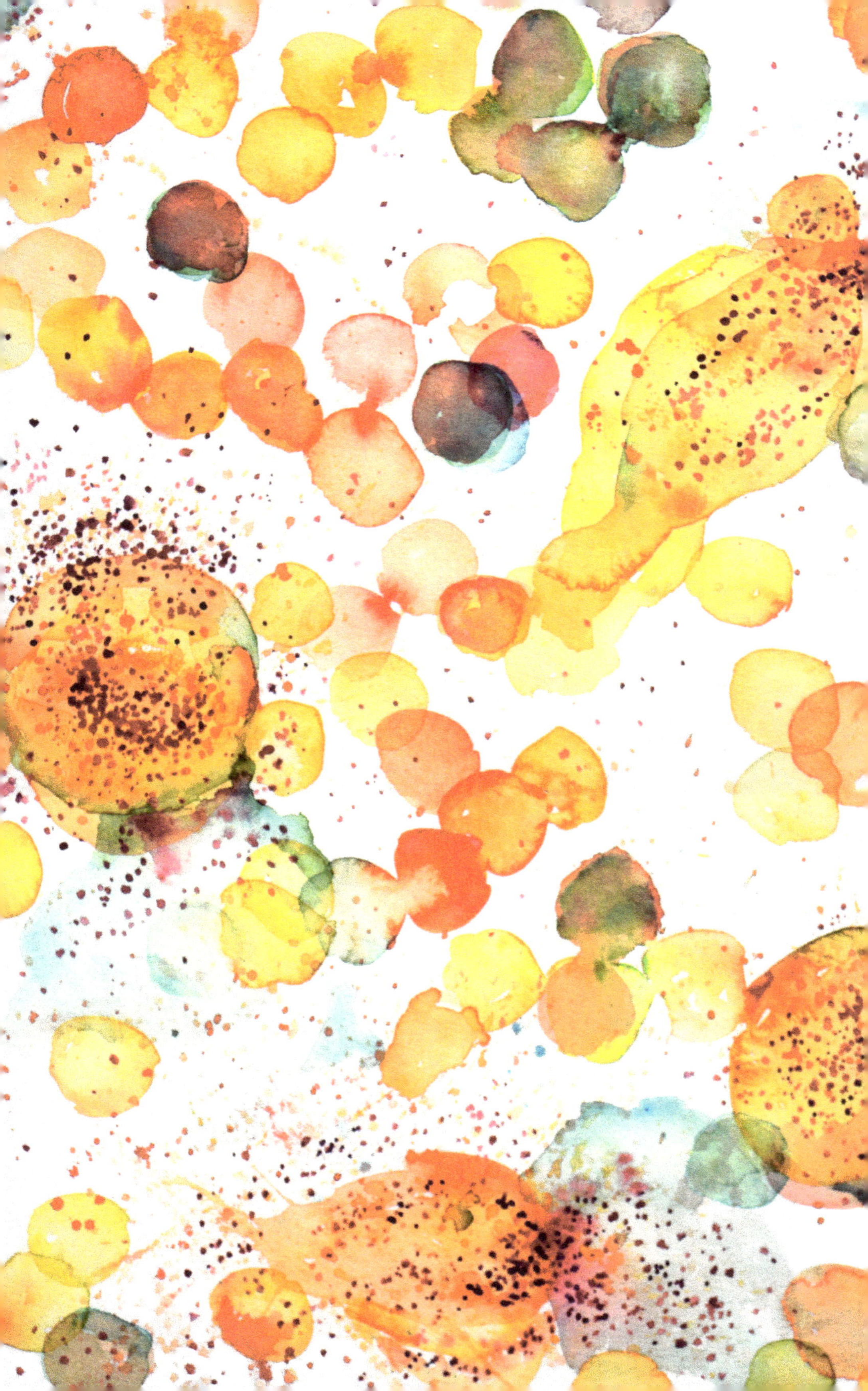

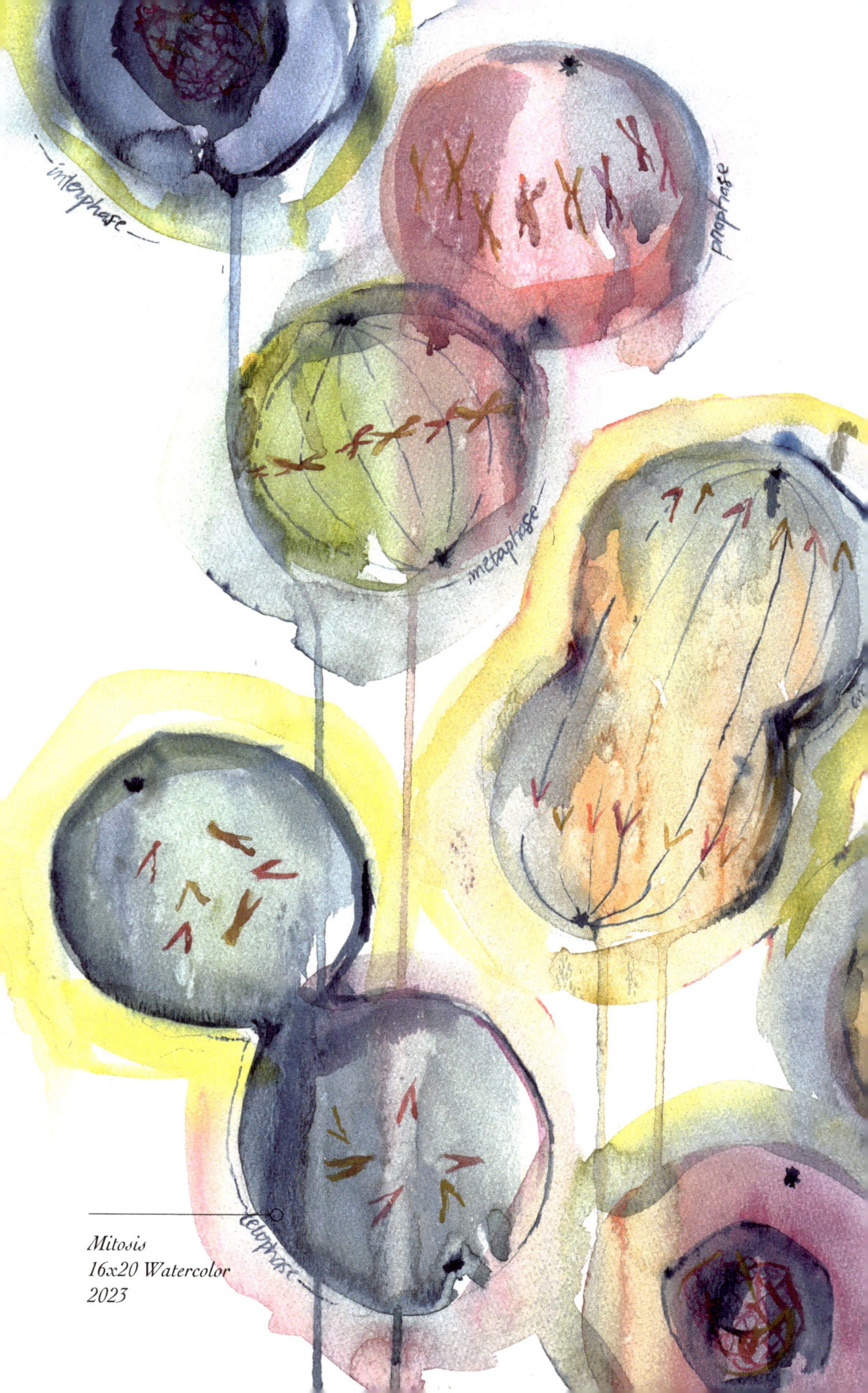

Mitosis
16x20 Watercolor
2023

O MITOSIS

O Mitosis, thou dost occasion cell division
Delivering a bounty of two daughter cells
Ornate replicas with no genetic revisions.

O Prophase, thou launches this process well,
Condensing chromosomes into neat visibility
While to the nucleolus thou bids farewell.

O Prometaphase, thou destroys the durability
Of the nuclear envelope, thus releasing all
The chromosomes within the facility.

O Metaphase, thy spindles answer thy call
To capture the chromosome population,
By attaching to each little kinetochore ball.

O Anaphase, portent of chromatid separation,
Twin sisters wrenched apart with a flare
By a smooth and steady microtubule operation.

O Telophase, thou marks an end to the affair,
The spindle breaks and two nuclei appear
And chromosomes unwind into strands of hair.

O Cytokinesis, thy actions also occur here,
When thy cytoplasm stretches and furrows,
And finally cleaves into twin daughter spheres.

O Mitosis, I appreciate thy process so thorough,
For within thee our longevity doth burrows.

SIX BLOOD CELLS

ONE is a lymphocyte
Whose antibodies take flight
To kill infections at first sight.
TWO is a monocyte
Who sees a dead cell's plight
So consumes it in a bite.
THREE, a neutrophil just might
Be the hero of the night
As first to the foreign body fight.
Eosinophil is FOUR, that's right,
The bane of the loathsome parasite,
Inducing inflammation with delight
(But can induce an allergy blight).
FIVE, the basophil is also quite
Involved in all of that allergy shite,
But also helps asthmatics see light.
And SIX, the red blood cell, so polite,
A battle he will never incite.
He's the one that's red, not white,
Sometimes dull, sometimes bright,
Relative to the oxygen on-site.

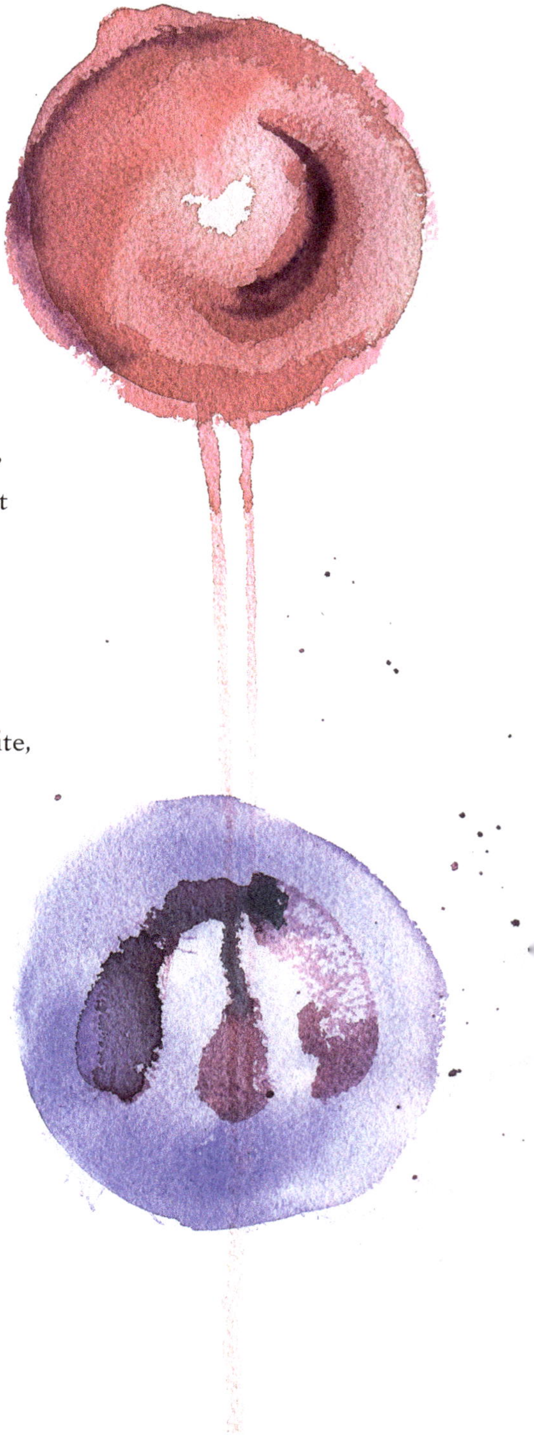

Six Blood Cells
20x16 Watercolor
2019

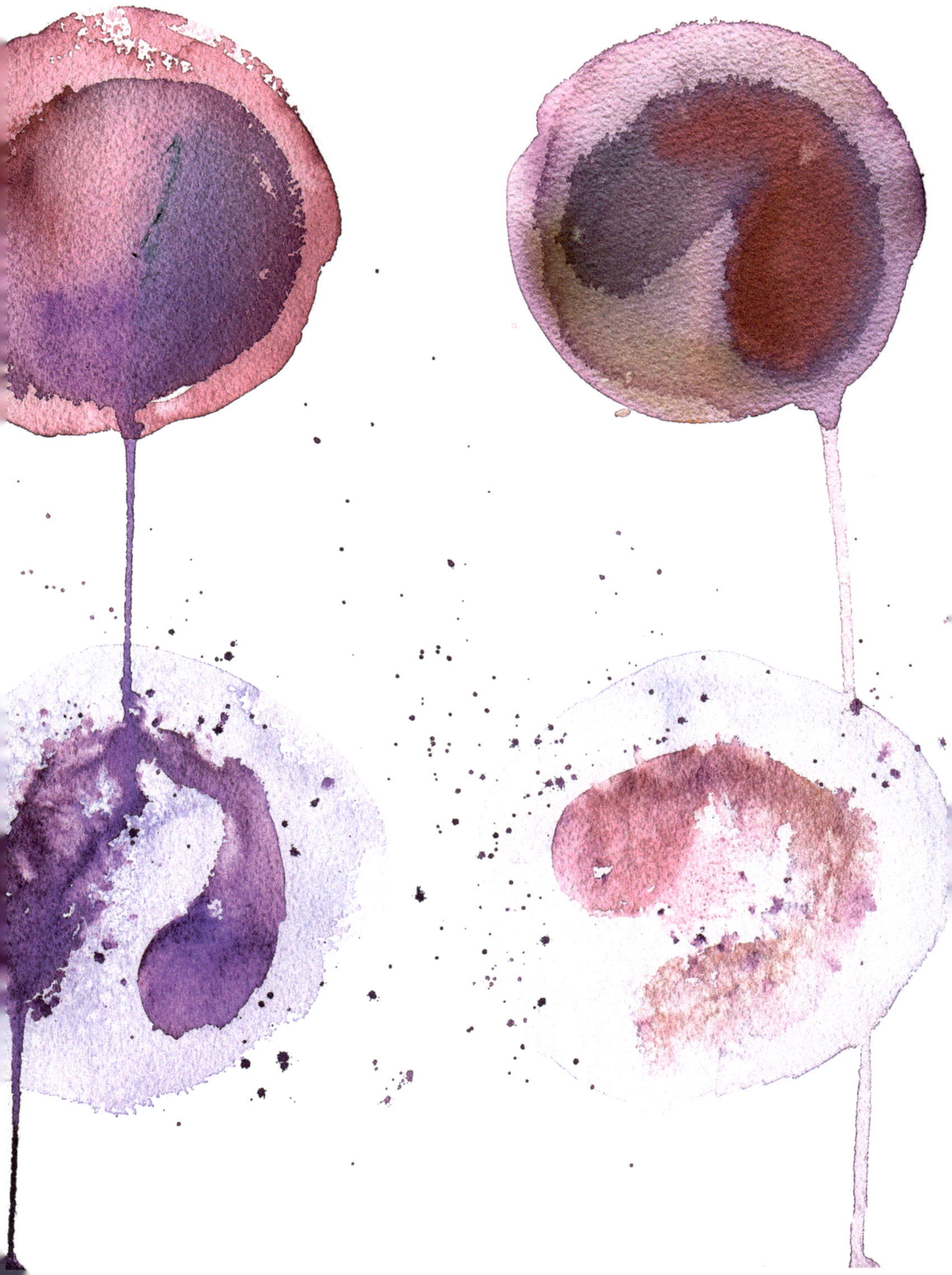

THE BALLAD OF THE CELL

Replicating its way into life,
A bold and curious cell
Awakens to find his sphere was rife
With functioning organelles.

Humming and working,
moving and jerking,
They ran like a well-run circus.
But as the cell took stock,
a thought began lurking…
"What is my overall purpose?"

That concern took hold like an
invading cancer:
"What oh what am I meant to be?"
He thought, "Organelles may
hold the answer!
"I'll look and then maybe I'll see."

A spherical stack caught his eye,
Like a heap of hollow pancakes.
It was the Golgi Body,
ruling the supply
Of all the protein and lipid flakes.

But his soul wasn't sparked,
so he moved on,
To a quivering bean of energy.
The ATP-making mitochondrion,
Who prevents cellular lethargy.

"I must learn more,
for he seemed fun!"
But then something else
caught his gaze.
It was the endoplasmic reticulum,
That monstrous, winding maze.

With regions ranging from
smooth to rough,
That labyrinth was infamous
For transporting around a
host of stuff,
And protein/lipid synthesis.

A simpler shape the cell next faced,
An undulating bubble.
'Twas the vacuole that eats all waste
Before it becomes trouble.

"You seem fine,
but you're not my guy,"
He said rather testily.
So with a sigh, he rolled on by,
Still dreaming of his destiny.

Onward he roamed until he strode
Up to a ball exuding power.
Filled with hope,
just one thought glowed:
"This must be my hour!"

"Nucleus, oh nucleus,
with just one glance,
"I knew you were so smart!
"Please oh please
just give me a chance:
My future, please do impart!"

"It's been just four weeks,
young cell, so wait!"
The nucleus said with asperity.
"For soon you'll start
to differentiate,
"And then you'll gain some clarity."

"But I'll give you hint to stop
you spinning"
Said the nucleus with rationality.
"Look to your membrane
to see the beginning
Of some individuality"

With a gasp, the cell turned to stare
At the rippling cellular floor,
Where he found a channel
he could swear
Hadn't been there before.

His mind a-wriggling,
his senses tingling,
He saw more outcroppings appear.
Branches grew out
and started mingling
With other cells that were near.

Then with a rumble,
the largest-yet tunnel
Burst forth into the night.
And when pillowy
myelin hugged the funnel,
The cell knew it was a dendrite.

"My fate's been decided,
and I am delighted!"
He sang to the ringing of bells.
"I am so lucky to have been invited
To be a noble neuron cell!"

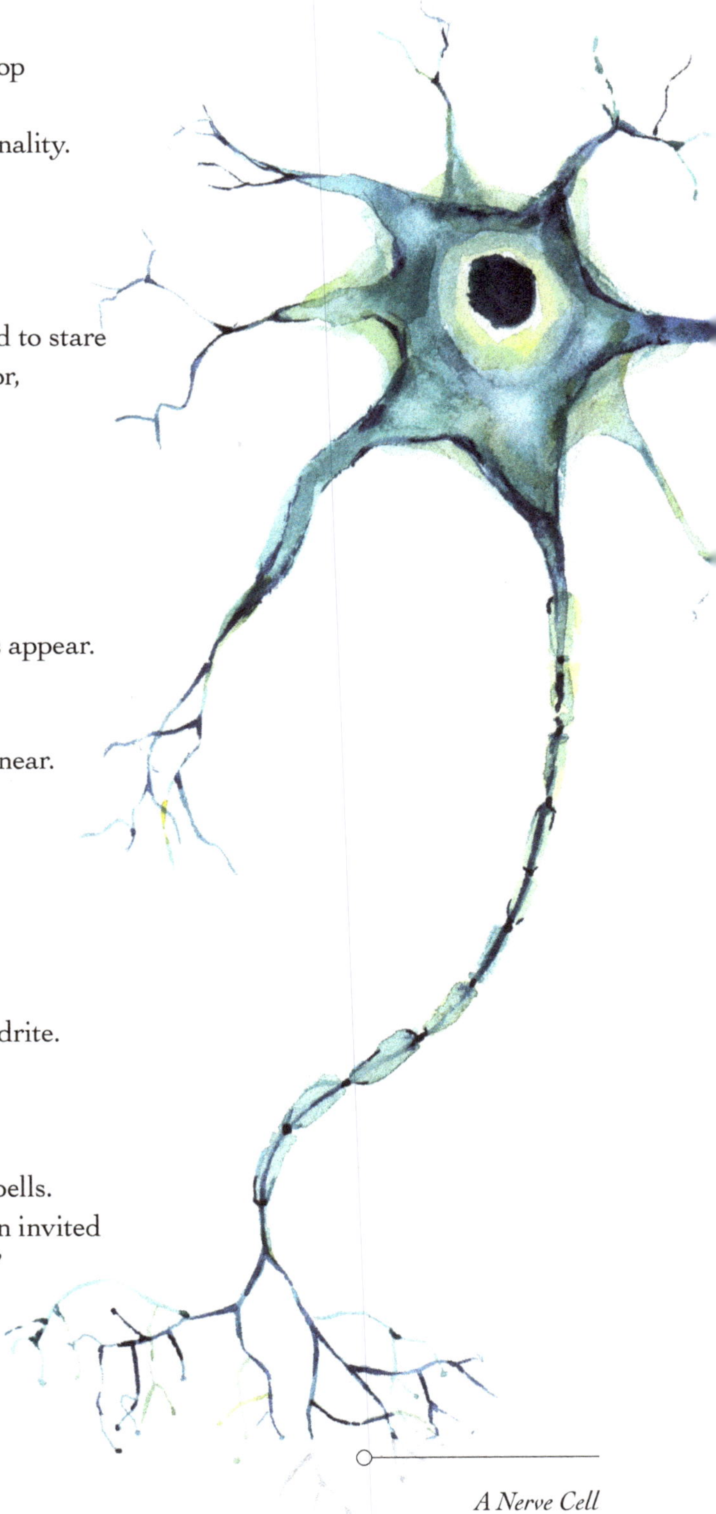

A Nerve Cell
9x12 Watercolor
2021

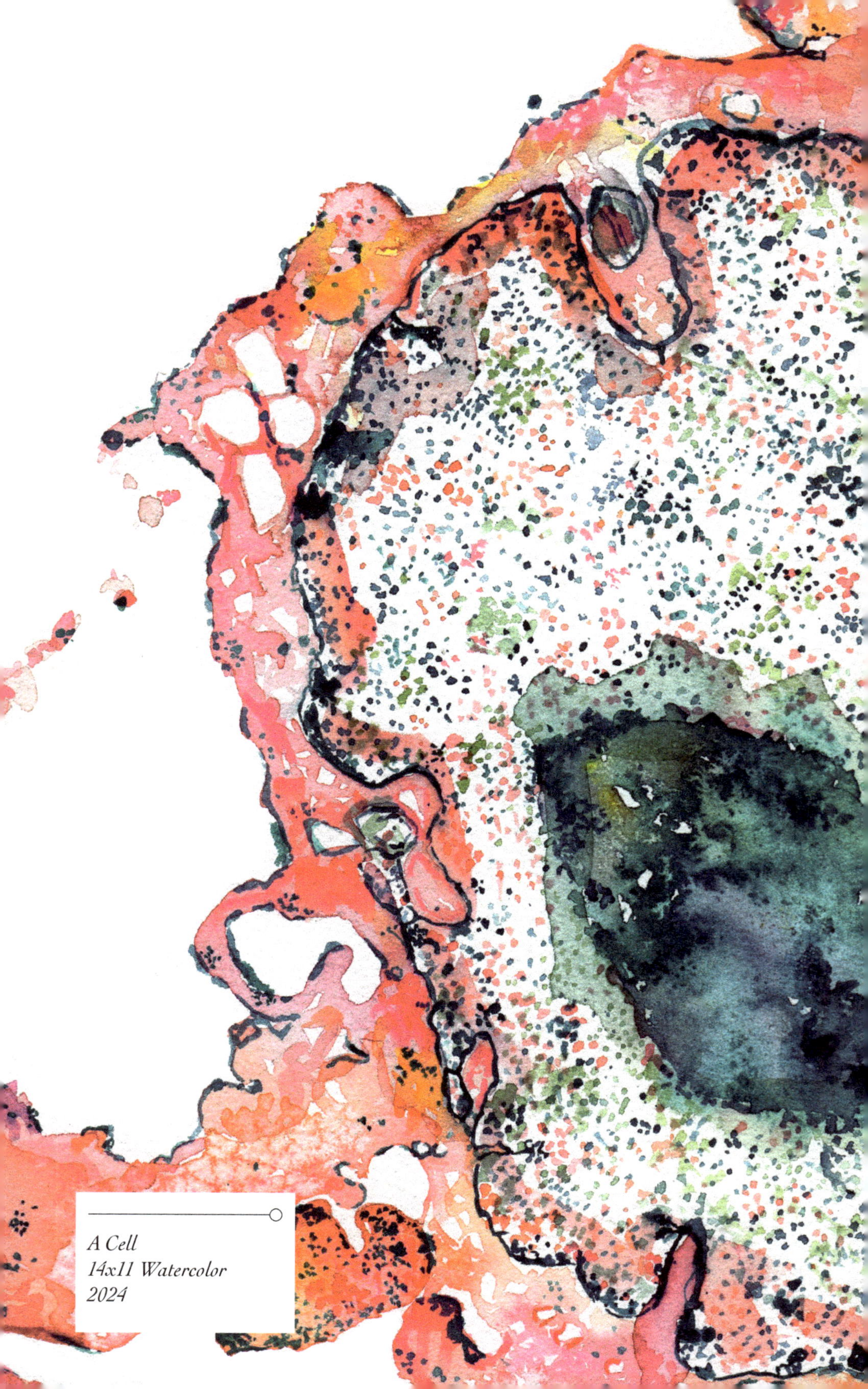

A Cell
14x11 Watercolor
2024

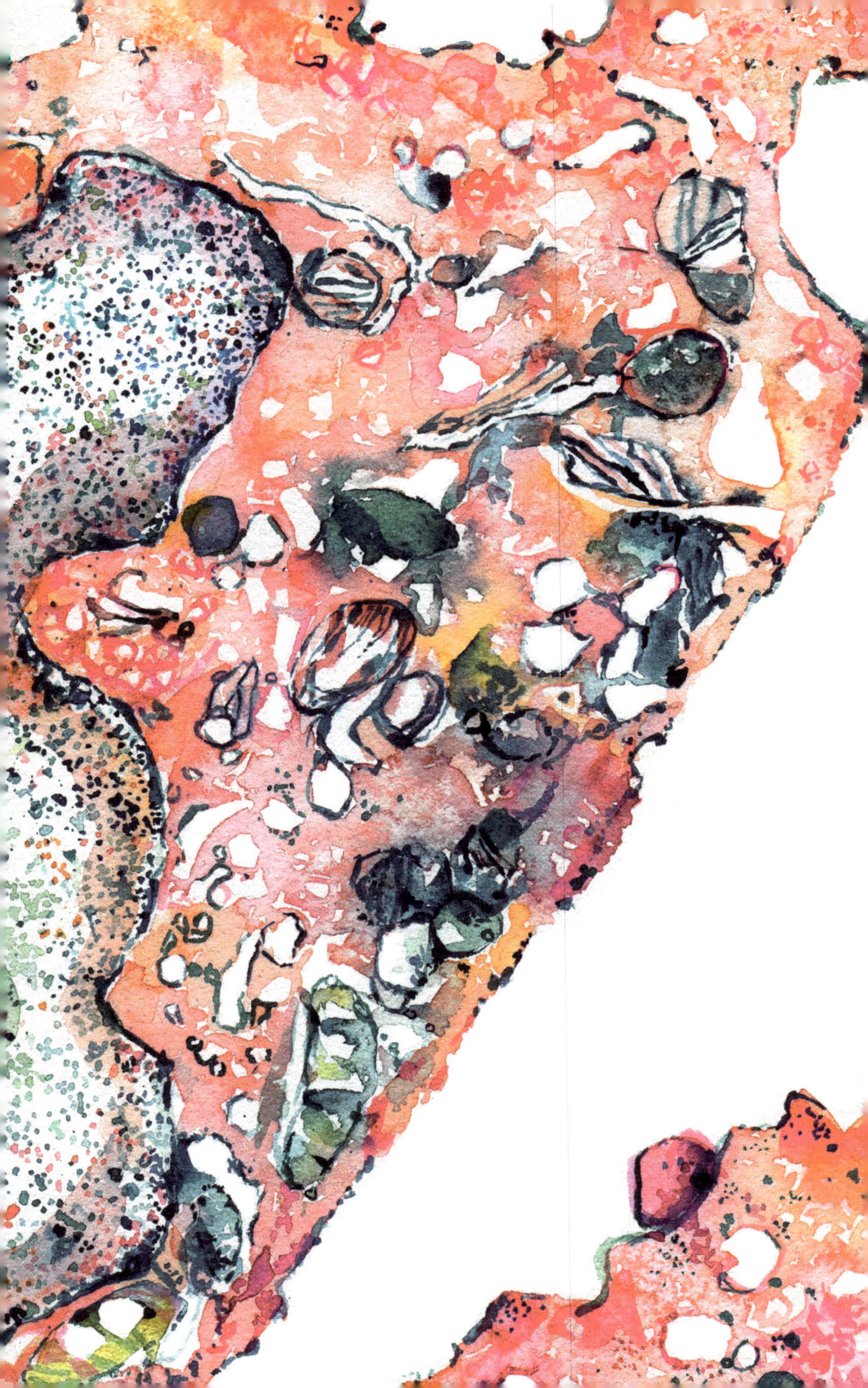

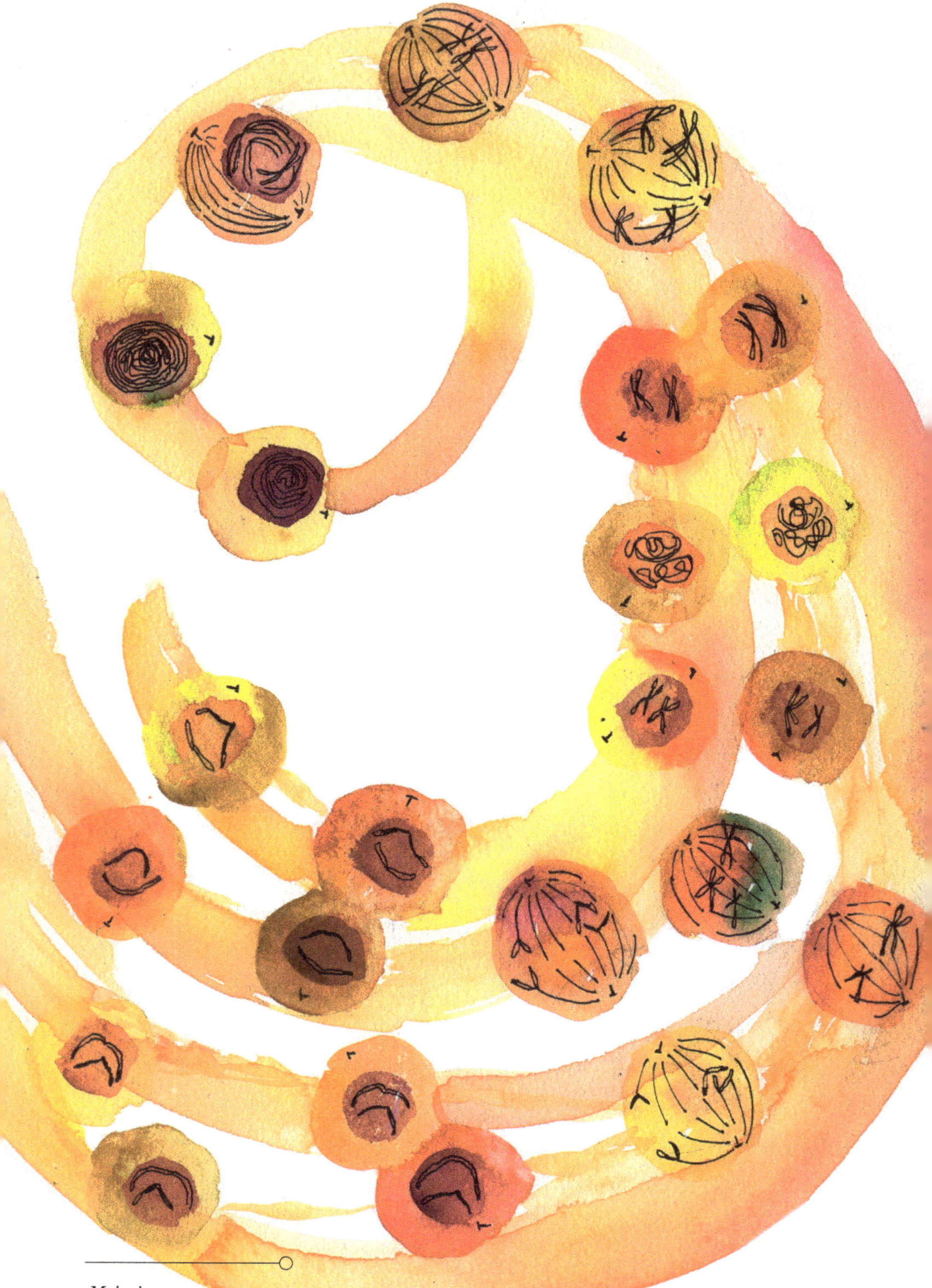

Meiosis
11x14 Watercolor
2024

O MEIOSIS

O meiosis, intrepid process for population renewal
Thou takes a cell and cleaves it to four,
Arming each with life's genetic fuel.

Thy journey embarks with prophase and more:
As chromosomes condense, an attraction incurs
Amongst pairs homologous, that they can't ignore.

Bound together, a swap occurs:
Chromosomes switch during recombination,
A parental DNA mix, from both his and from hers.

Thy next duty lies in chromosomal organization
With homologous pairs on a metaphase plate,
Then pulled by microtubules in opposite locations.

Next thou sails through the divisional states
Ending post-telophase with two cells so fresh.
Each with all their chromosomes — but wait!

Gamete cells need but half, for they mesh
Together with other cells during sex,
Joining up chromosomes, after flesh meets flesh.

O thou art clever and wise for what thou does next,
Enacting a second round of divisional phases,
But with none of the DNA replication effects.

O Meiosis, thou dost earn our unending praises,
For the four granddaughter cells thou dost raises.

THE IN-BETWEEN

Mysterious as a druid,
The interstitial fluid
Is the undisputed steward
   Of the in-between.

It resides not in a cell,
Ignores the blood as well,
Instead chooses to dwell
   Amongst the in-between.

For a tissue's refurbishment,
It needs no encouragement
To carry the nourishment
   Through the in-between.

Nimble as a nymph,
Leaping from skiff to skiff,
Until it turns to lymph,
   No longer in-between.

Interstitial Fluid
9x12 Watercolor & Alcohol Ink on Yupo
2024

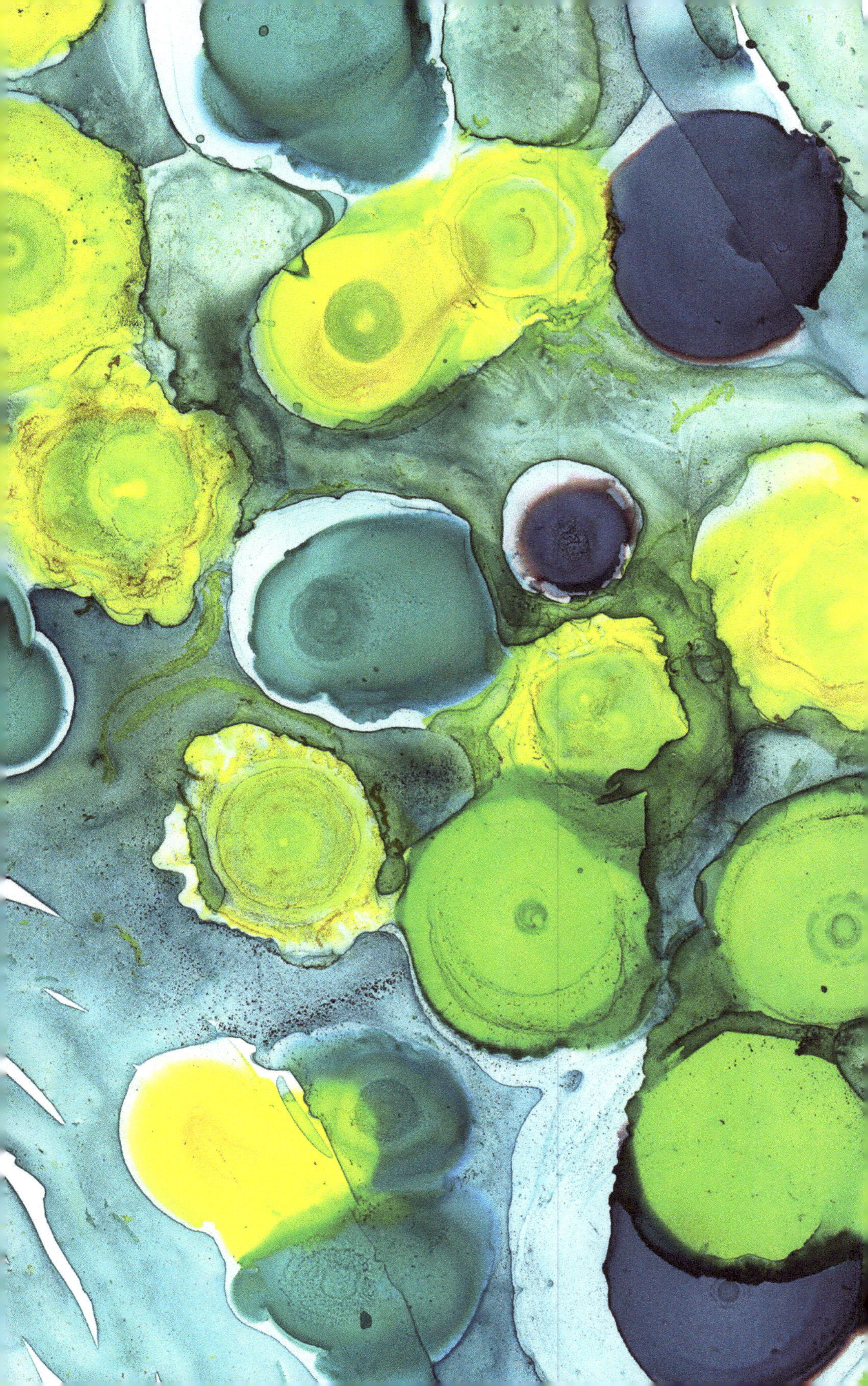

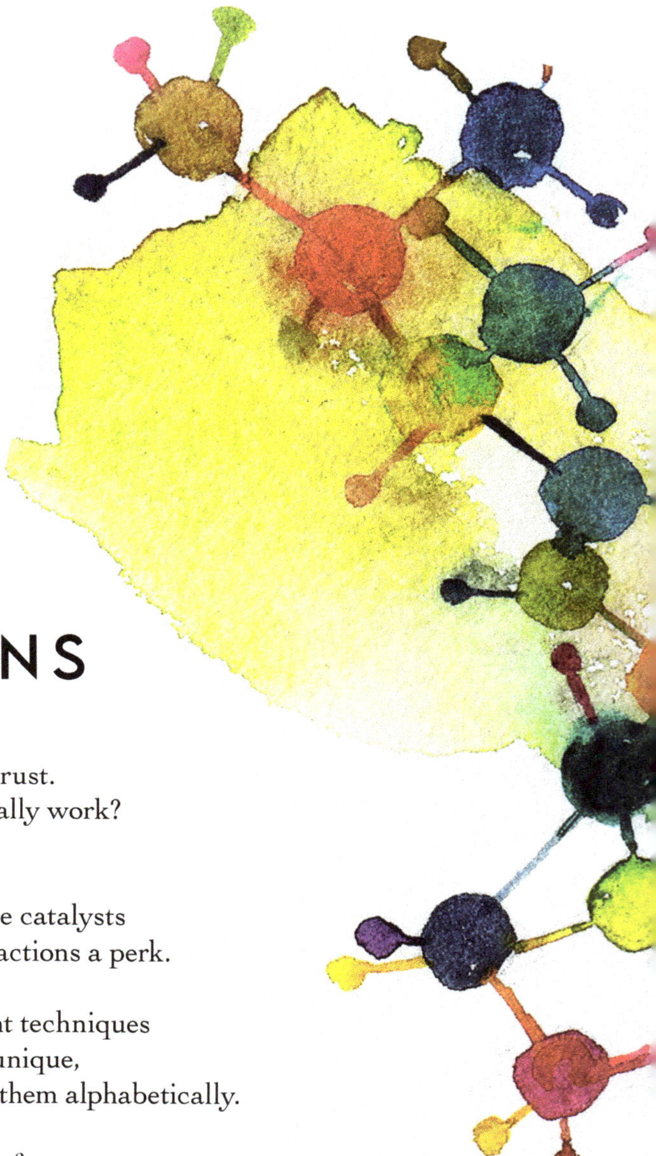

VITAMINS

Vitamins are a must!
Say all the moms we trust.
But how do they actually work?

After some analysis
I see their enzymes are catalysts
That give chemical reactions a perk.

But each uses different techniques
And their effects are unique,
So let's walk through them alphabetically.

Improving the health of your eyes,
Plus the immune and reproductive guys,
Vitamin A does most energetically.

Vitamin Bs are actually a gang
Of chemicals that all aid
Cell metabolism and RBC production.

B12 in particular is renown,
To help those sad, sluggish or down,
Providing you with energy to function.

Next up is Vitamin C,
The immune system's Queen Bee,
And an antioxidant of great import.

Vitamin D gives bones an assist
When it absorbs the calcium missed,
While also giving good mood support.

E gives free radicals the boot
As an antioxidant brute,
While it also quenches the skin.

Then we jump to Vitamin K
Who helps with healing all day
By causing clots to form within.

And that there is a start
To vitamins that do their part,
Keeping your health not so shoddy.

I encourage you to learn them all,
But even if they don't enthrall,
Do try to put them in your body!

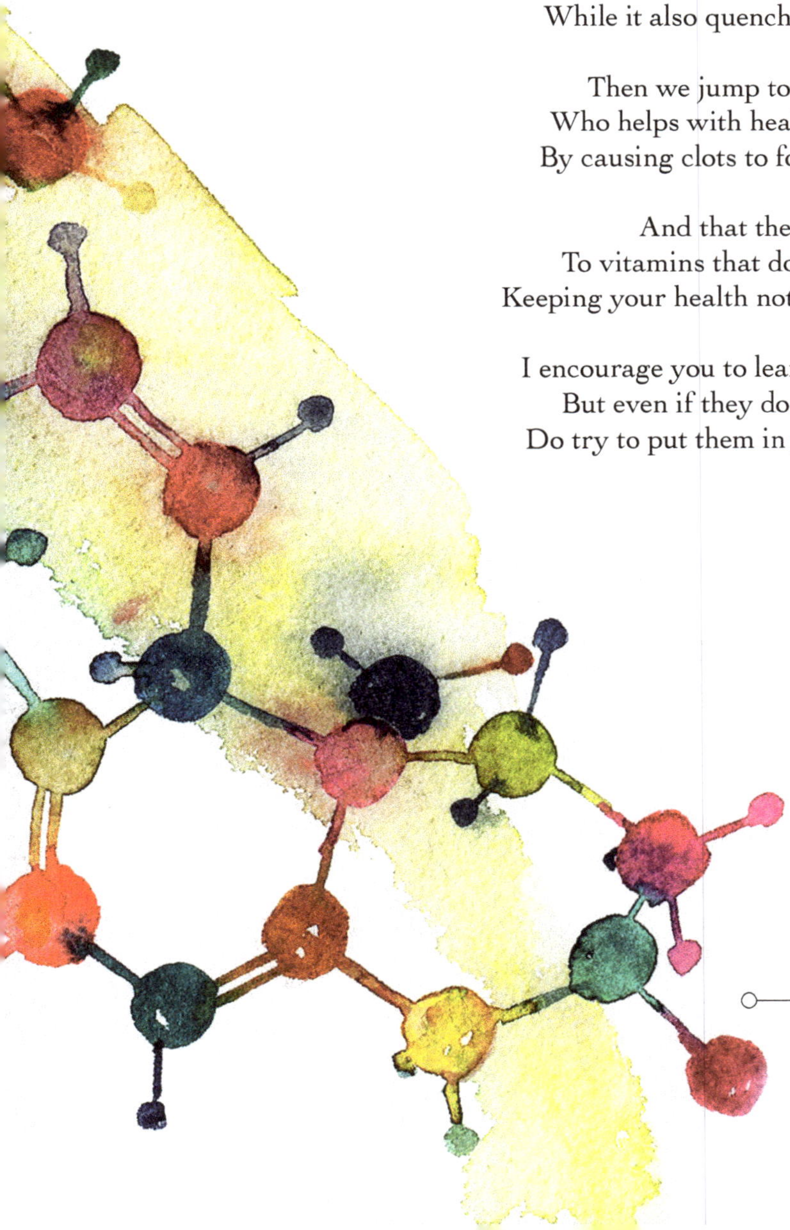

Vitamin D
6x9 Watercolor
2024

MOODY

The lack of serotonin's
Got me mean and moanin.
I feel cranky and not bright
So this is all I'm going to write.

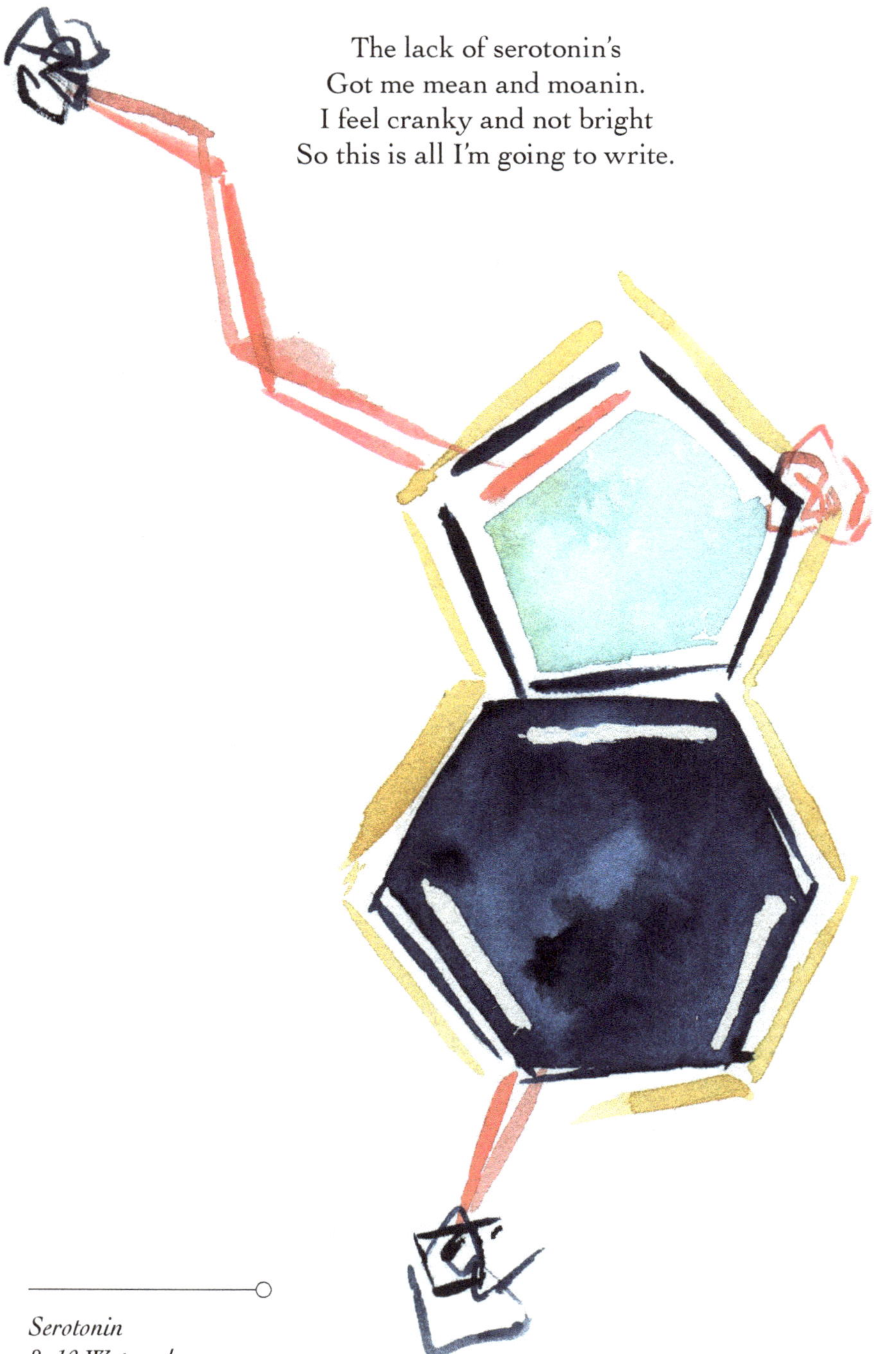

Serotonin
8x10 Watercolor
2020

chapter three

BRAIN & NERVE THINGS

"All our knowledge has its origins in our perceptions."

-Leonardo Da Vinci

Brain Stem
8x10 Watercolor
2024

HANS THE PONS

Hans the Pons, the bloke with connections
Carries messages in all directions.
From the main brain he receives a collection
Of signals to take to two sections:
He delivers to the medulla with affection
As well as to that cerebellum confection.
He also transfers the sensory impressions
To the thalamus for their inspection.
Hans the Pons, the bloke with connections
A key player in the brain delivery profession.

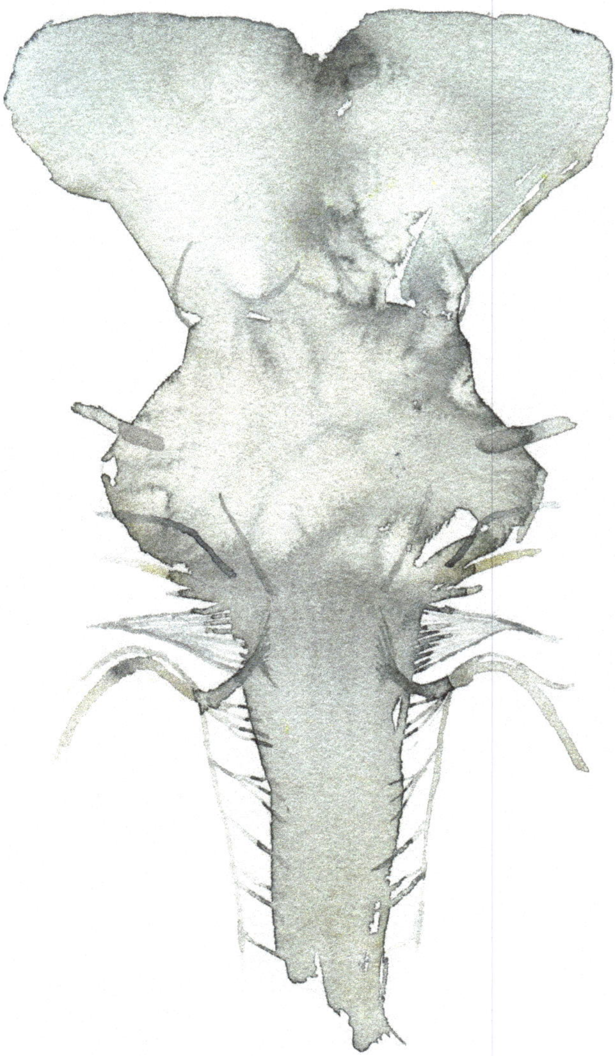

CRANIAL NERVES

Olfactory
is sensory
And lets you smell the flowers.

Optic nerve
Helps you observe
'Cause vision is her power.

Oculomotor,
A blink's promoter,
And boss of that pupil hole.

The trochlear dude
Has attitude
'Cause he helps your eyes roll.

Trigeminal
Of himself he's full
Because he has three branches
He does do much
With motor and touch.
(That's why he gets more stanzas).
With him a face feels
And you can chew meals
So I guess he's earned my praise.

Compared to his fame
Abducen's quite lame
The eyes he only shifts sideways.

Facial can taste
And she innervates
Muscles of facial expression.

Vestibulocochlear
Allows you to hear
And has a balance obsession.

Glossopharyngeal
Lets you move and feel
The throat and tongue in the back.

The diverse Vagus
Is quite famous,
Keeping visceral organs on track.

Ms. Accessory
Gets the glory
For moving the shoulder and neck.

Hypoglossal,
The tongue he jostles,
Making its movements complex.

The Cranial Nerves
16x20 Watercolor
2019

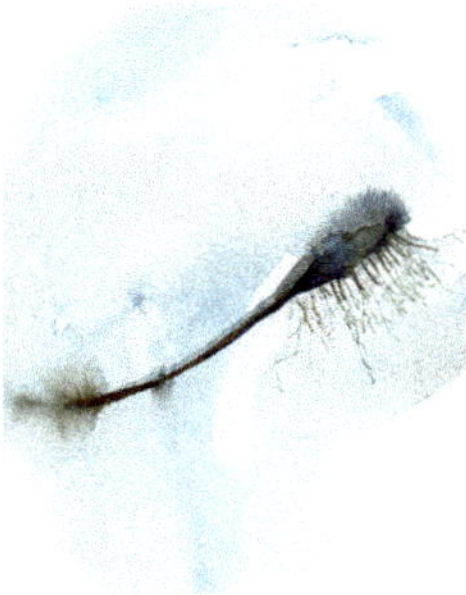

i. olfactory

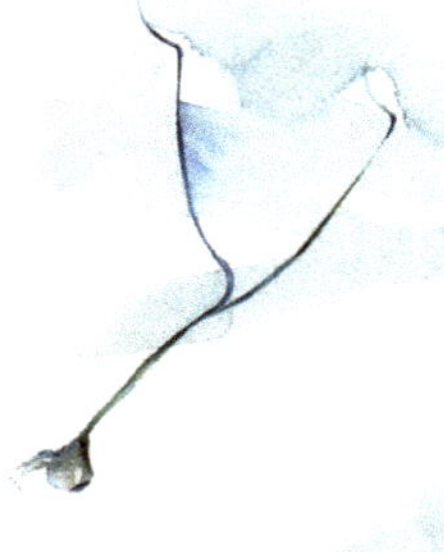

ii optic

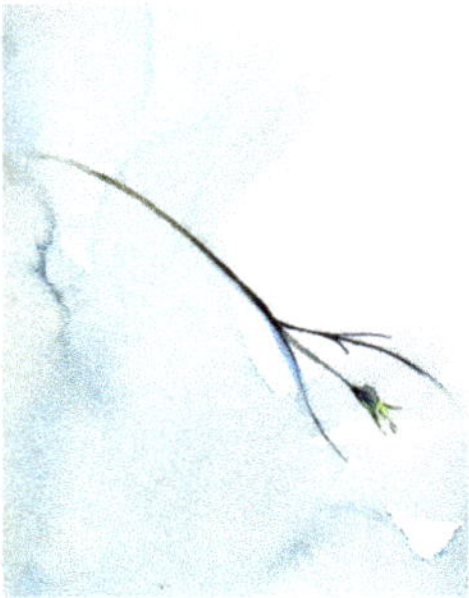

iii oculomotor

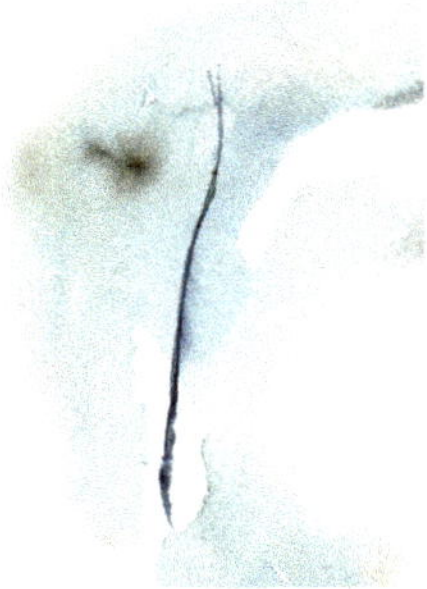

iv. trochlear

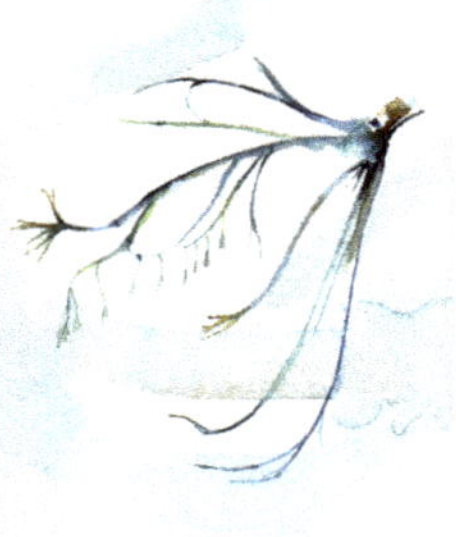

v. trigeminal

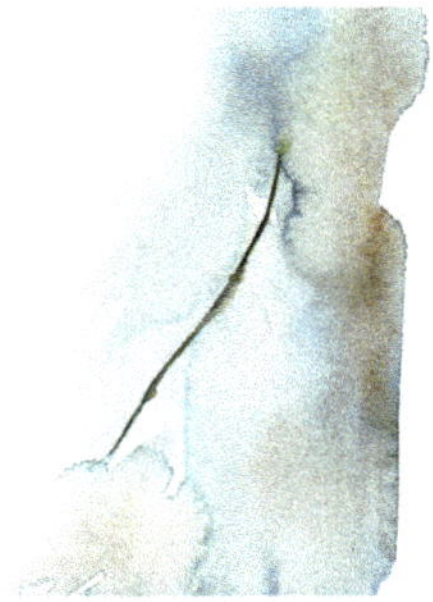

vi. abducens

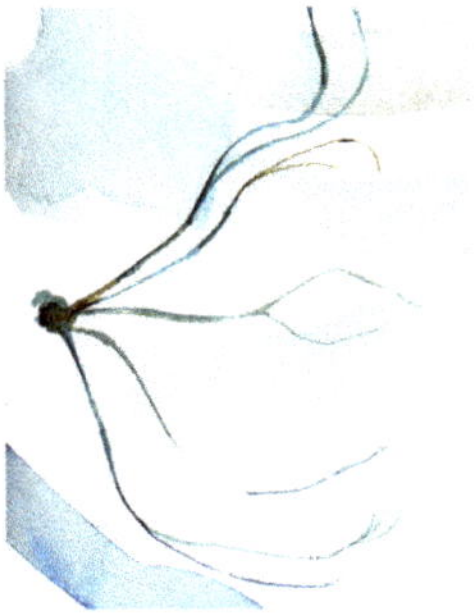

vii. facial

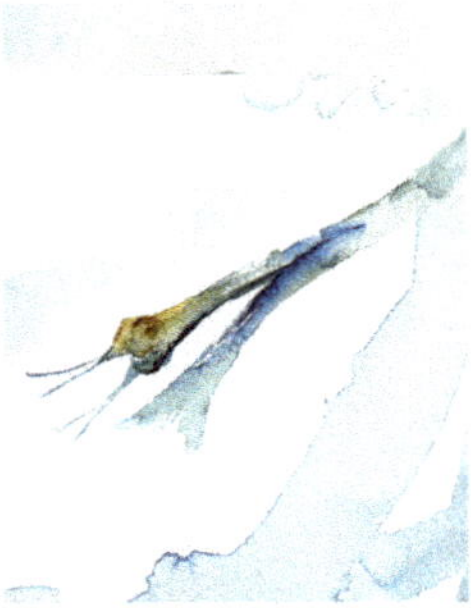

viii. vestibulocochlear

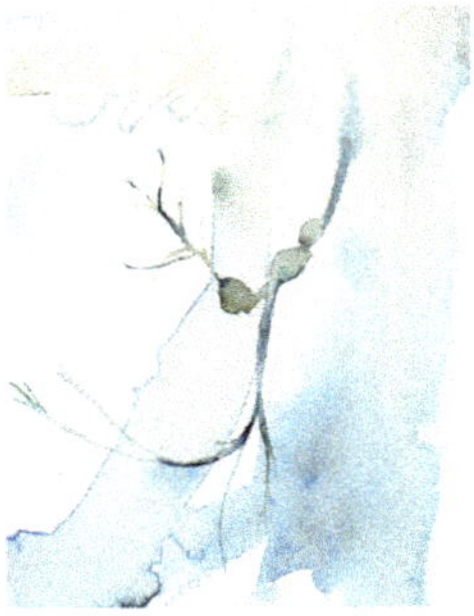

ix. glossopharyngeal

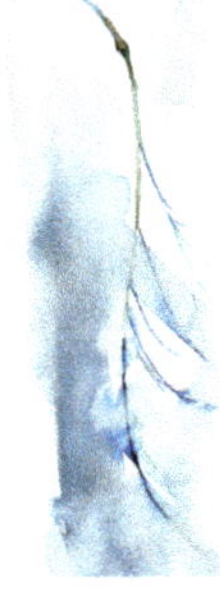

x. vagus

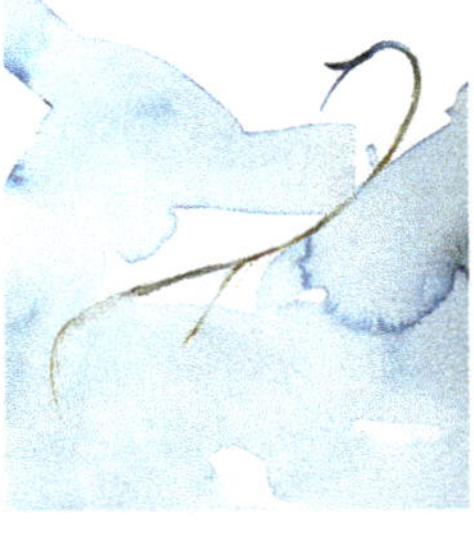

xi. accessory

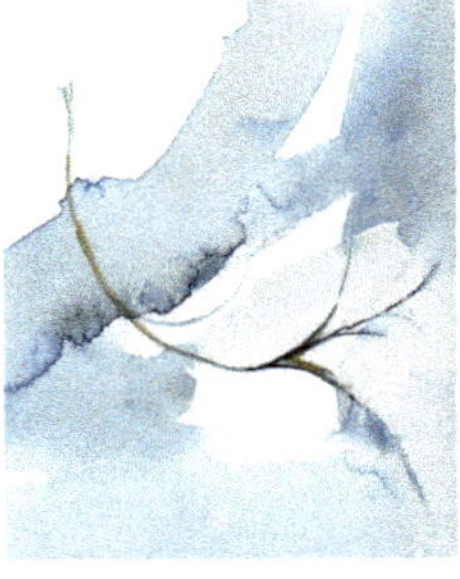

xii. hypoglossal

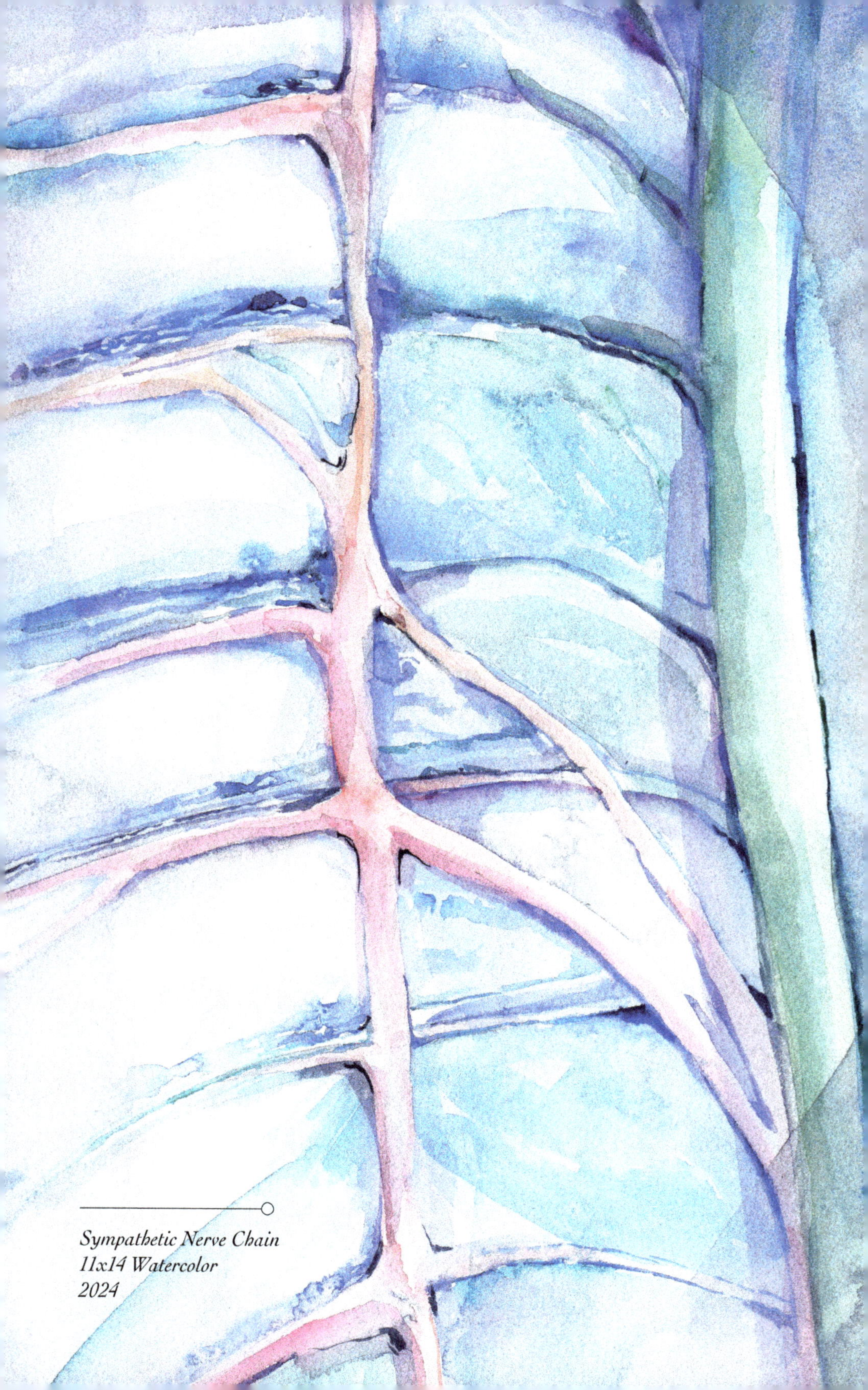

Sympathetic Nerve Chain
11x14 Watercolor
2024

SYMPATHETIC NERVE CHAIN

Chugga-chugga chugga-chugga choo choo...
We nerve impulses are on a ride.
Along these chains we slide
From the skull, and down to the coccyx too!

Clackety-clack, we cruise two tracks...
On both sides of the spine we sway,
Observing the vertebrae,
Until we're ready to make an impact!

From the body we brought information
And zoomed till we landed on
A paravertebral ganglion
And swapped news at this relay station.

Wheee! Some afferent fibers carry us out
Then up to the brain we head
Via rami communicantes threads
"DANGER! DANGER!" we finally shout!

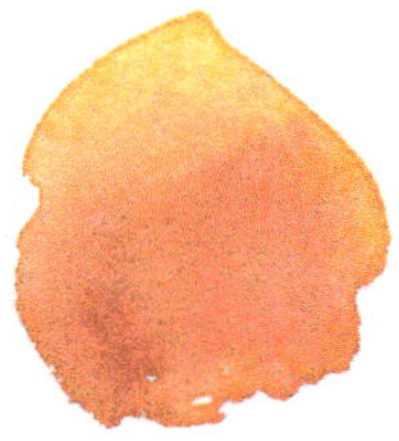

AMYGDALA

You know what is an enigma?
The intriguing little amygdala.
That beguiling nuclei cluster,
What strong emotion it musters.
A trove of intense feeling
That sometimes leave you reeling.
For passion, anger and fear
Emanate from right here.
While its influence can be dramatic,
Leading to anxiety and panic,
Don't think of it as all wrong
For it can keep you safe and strong.
So my only tiny complaint?
It's too boring-looking to paint.

Amygdala Blob
4x4 Watercolor
2017

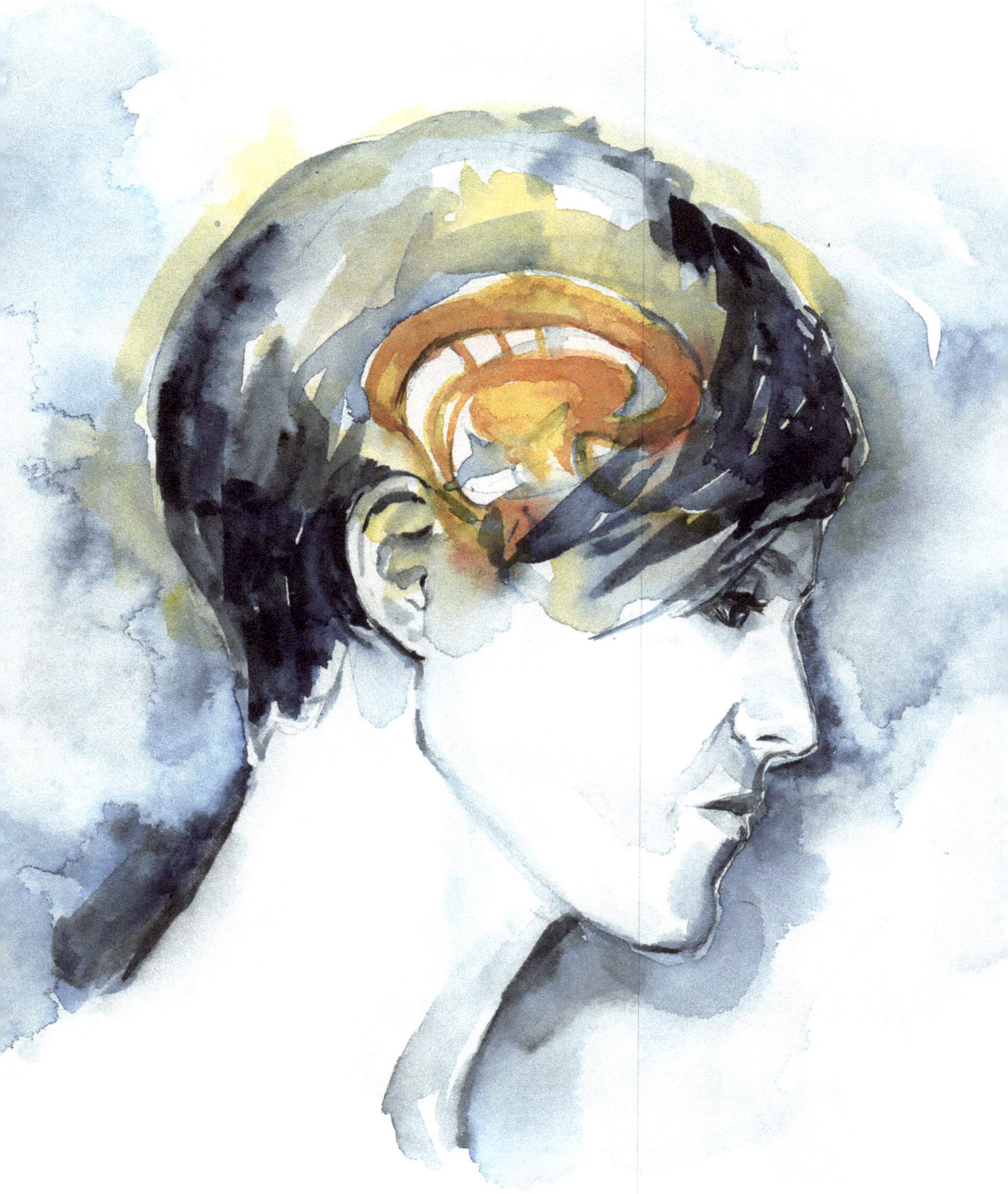

Limbic System
11x14 Watercolor
2020

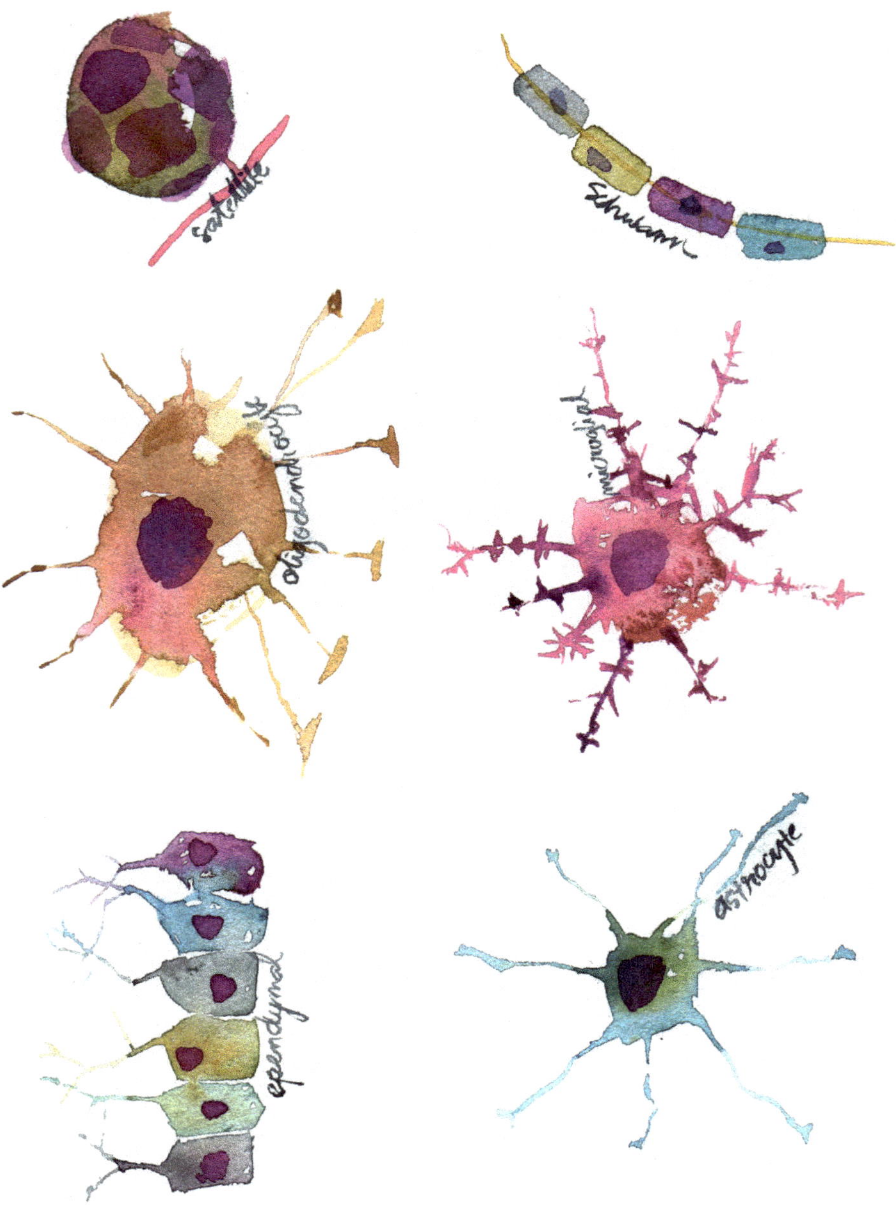
satellite
Schwann
oligodendrocyte
microglial
ependymal
astrocyte

GLIAL

Neurons have this reputation
For providing all the communication
Between the brain and everything else.

Taken in by their mysterious might,
Their spidersilk axons and dendrites,
A person's heart always melts.

But you know who does the real shit?
Who gets no credit, not even a bit?
Those of us referred to as glial.

We many not have an e-current,
But don't let that be a deterrent,
For the work we do is real.

Supporters, protectors and risk reducers,
Homeostasis guarders and myelin producers,
Our actions have an effect.

Schwann, satellite, oligodendrocytes
Ependymal, microglia, and astrocytes:
We all demand your respect!

Glial Cells
8x10 Watercolor
2024

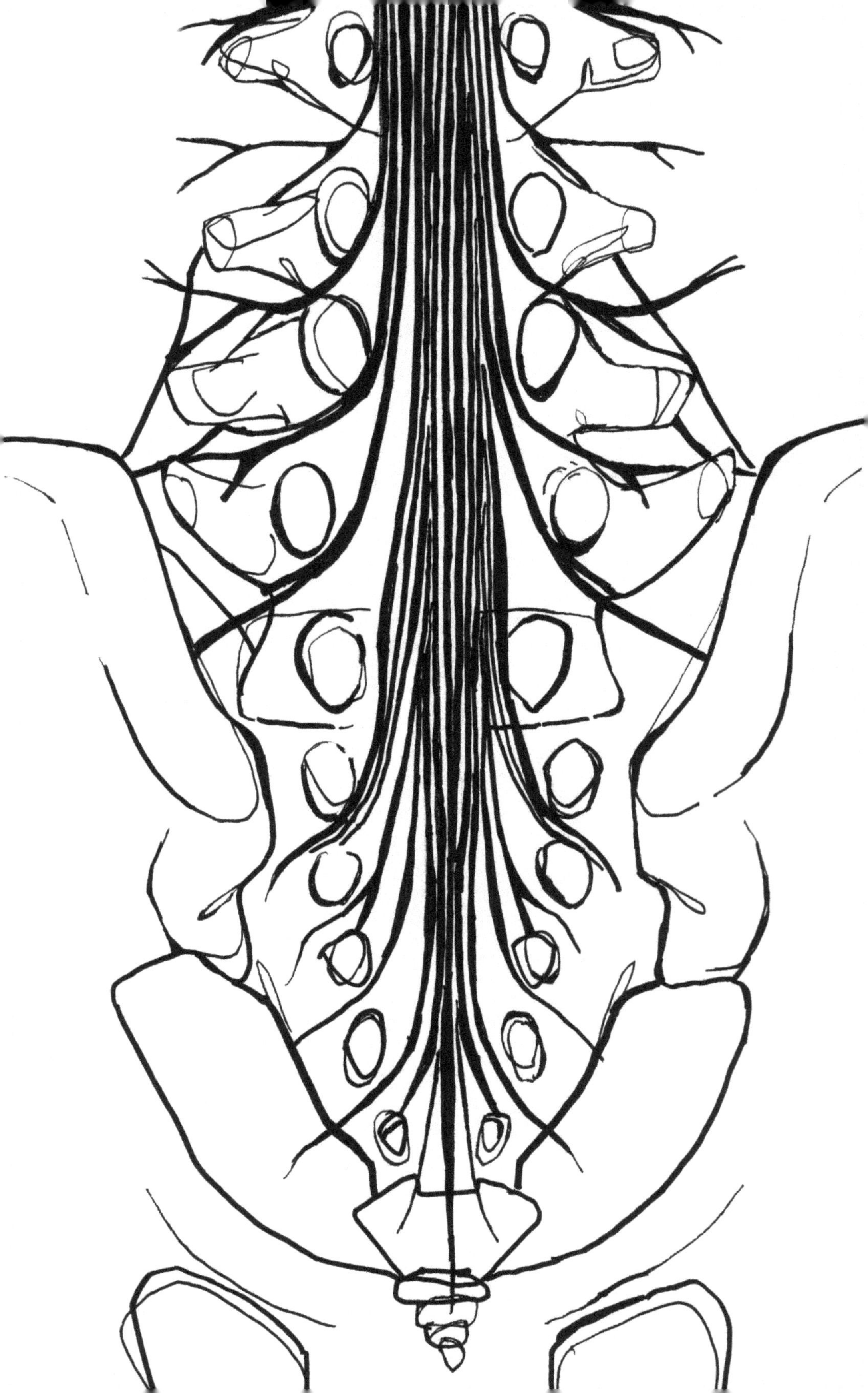

CAUDA EQUINA

Glossy, silver strands
That would slip through my hands.
Long and wispy tresses,
Made for gentle caresses.
Fibers elegantly trail
Like a horse's sprightly tail.
An elongated fringe
Provides an electric bridge.
For it's not hair my mind observes
But a bundle of trailing nerves.

Cauda Equina
10x16 Pen & Ink
2024

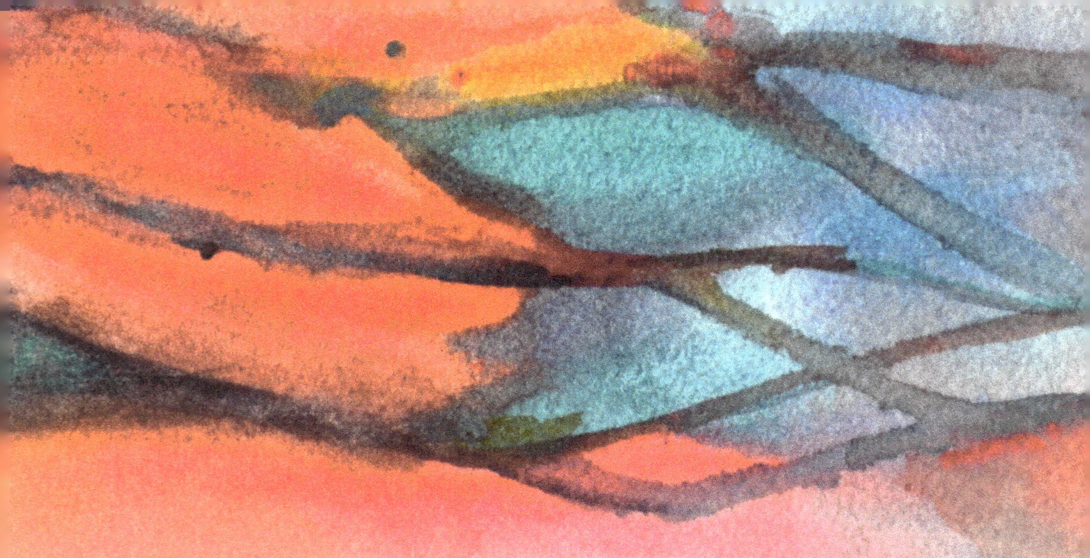

BRACHIAL PLEXUS

It's time to talk about the brachial plexus
Let's start at the top with the roots and trunk nexus.

A new nerve is formed by C5 and C6
The "superior trunk" we call them once mixed.

Poor C7, though, moves along all alone
And becomes the middle trunk all on its own.

(These three roots also toss you a swerve
As they each donate to the long thoracic nerve.)

The inferior trunk's made by C8 and T1.
Then the roots and trunks are already done!

Next, those three trunks all split with precision
Into an anterior and posterior division.

The posterior divisions of all three trunks
Combine into one large posterior cord hunk.

The anterior divisions are next on the griddle.
But only those made by trunks superior and middle.

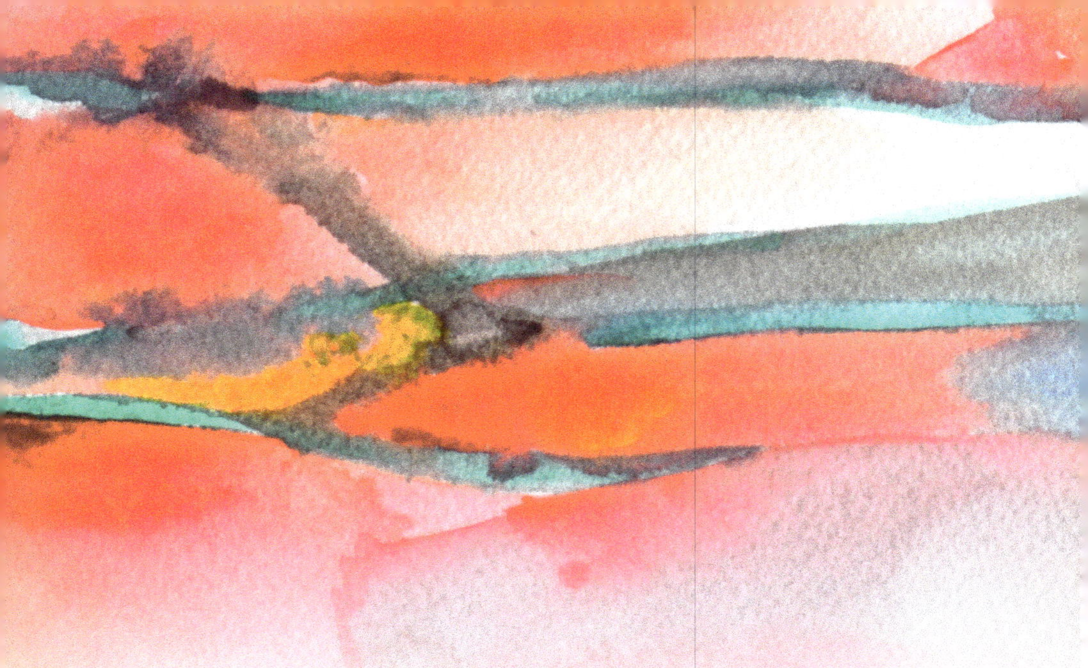

For just these two join in order to form
A brand new bundle named the lateral cord.

Last up is the inferior trunk's anterior split.
The medial cord is made by this lonely bit.

The cords are done, but don't disengage!
It's time for the branches to take center stage.

First, as the medial cord migrates on down
It becomes the ulnar nerve of renown.

The posterior cord has a transformation,
To radial, nerve of thumb operation.

The lateral cord likewise gets an alias.
It becomes known as musculocutaneous.

Medial and posterior cords also provide
Fibers to make that median nerve guy.

And with that we're done with the arm's nervy mess!
Now can I go home and perhaps take a rest?

Brrachial Plexus
19x15 Watercolor
2015

MY PATH TO SERENITY

My mind is pacing, my heart's racing for a reason I'm still waiting to appear.
I am manic and I'm frantic as I chase a finish line that disappears.

The world demands I ride or die on every task that I perform.
Or is it just me who wants to be it all and then a little more?

Regardless, it's not harmless, it causes me despair.
I seek peace but I can't seem to find it anywhere.

But friend, I've heard there's hope.
Within a parasympathetic rope.

If I can just learn to stimulate
And thoroughly invigorate

A nerve of innate calm
I'll unearth a steady balm.

That vagus nerve tree:
My path to serenity.

Vagus Nerve
11x14 Watercolor
2019

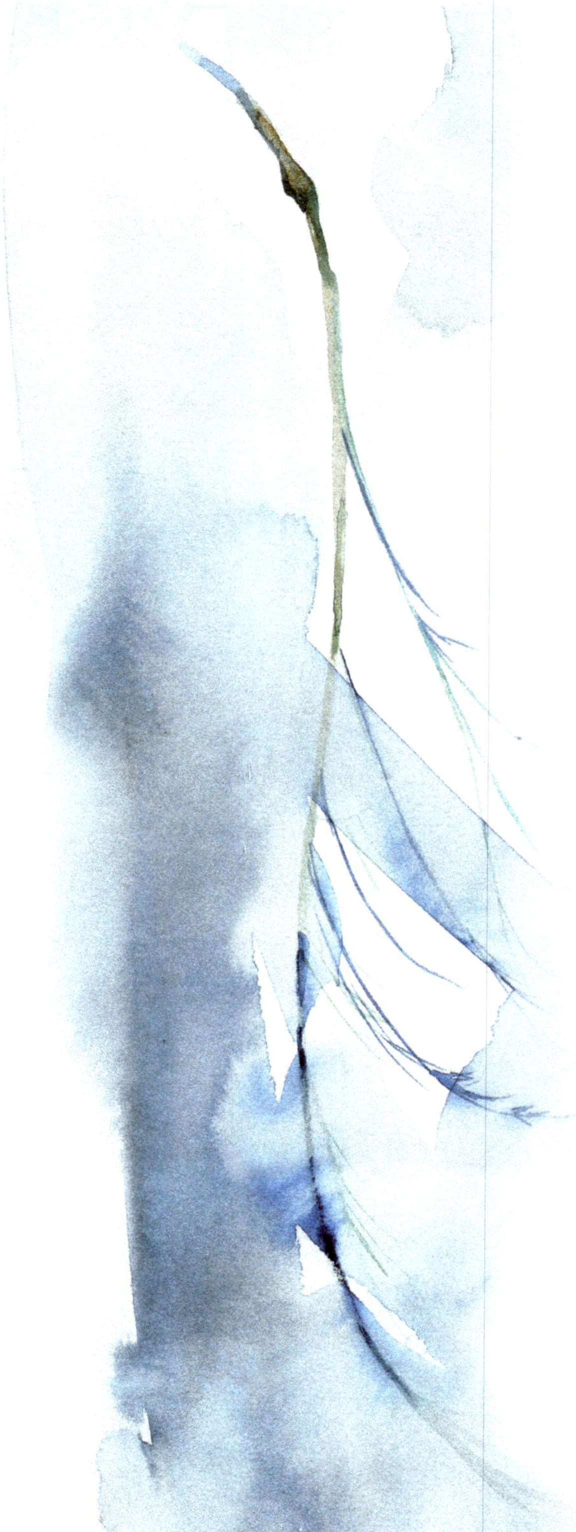

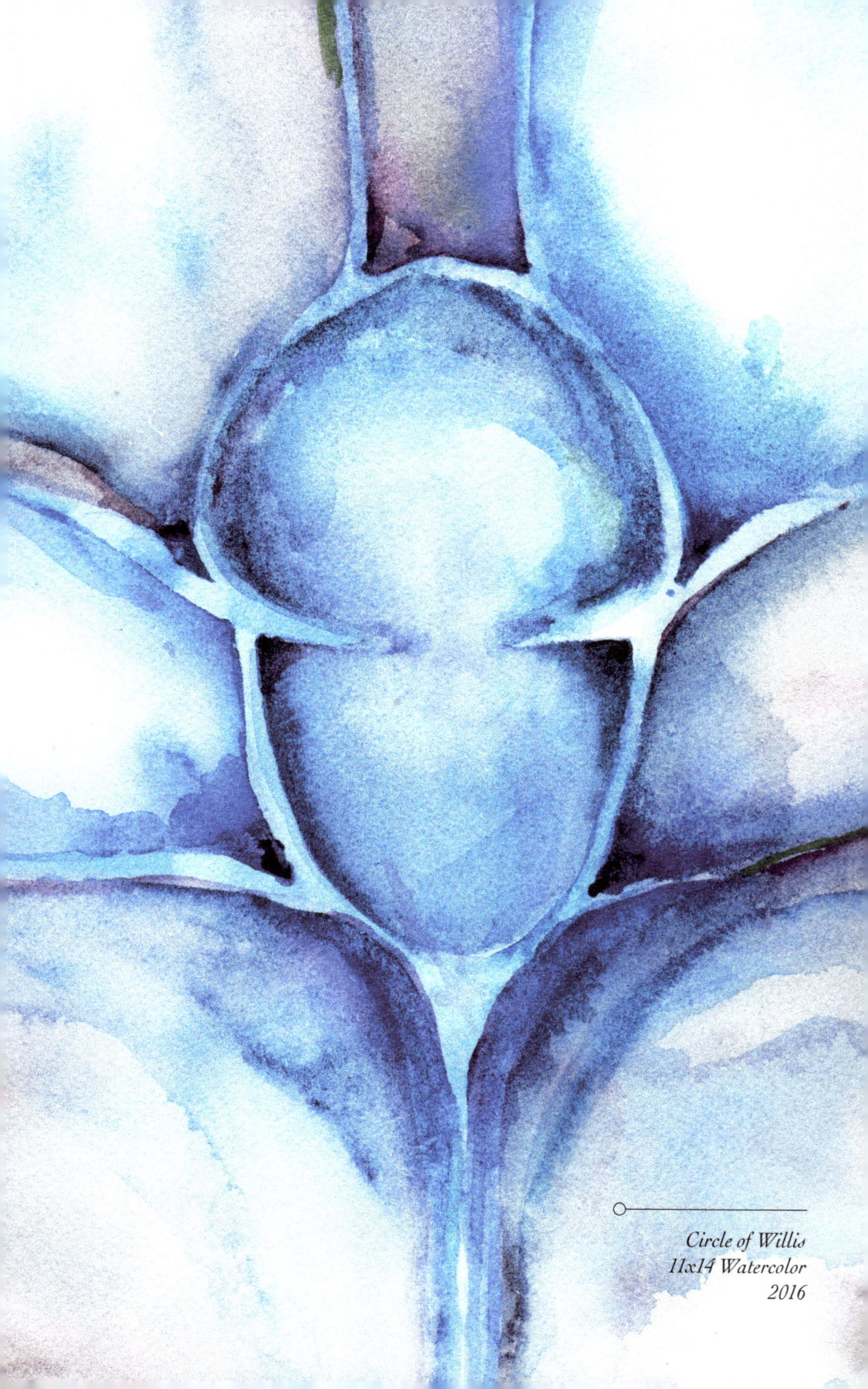

Circle of Willis
11x14 Watercolor
2016

CIRCLE OF WILLIS

Round and round the brain we go,
Bestowing an endless, crimson flow.

Blood rich with oxygen does fill us,
We arteries of the Circle of Willis.

Anterior communicating sets the tone
As it's out in front and on its own,

Joining anterior cerebrals, right and left
As they carry the blood to lobes bereft.

These intersect the internal carotids,
Up from the neck these both plodded.

Then come the posterior communicatings,
Who with the cerebrals does some mating

Including the last to round the bend,
The posterior cerebrals—the occipital's friend.

Round and round the brain we go,
Bestowing an endless, crimson flow.

BRAIN NAME EDUCATION

Without Wernicke's Area
There would be hysteria
Because we wouldn't understand speech.

The Circle of Willis
Won't stop until it's
Given blood to all structures in reach.

Corpus callosum
Is considered quite wholesome
Because it joins two brains.

Somatosensory cortex
Is a vortex
Of sensations like touch and pain.

In speech we invoke a
Region called Broca,
The brain's local scriptwriter.

The amygdala appears
To take on feels and fears.
And he can really be a fighter.

Medulla oblongata
Contains a whole lotta
Nerves signals from the spine.

The diencephalon
Holds a salon
For autonomic control shrines.

The cingulate gyrus
Is good in a crisis,
As it does behavior regulation.

And now thanks to me,
You're a doctor basically,
Ready to do a brain operation.

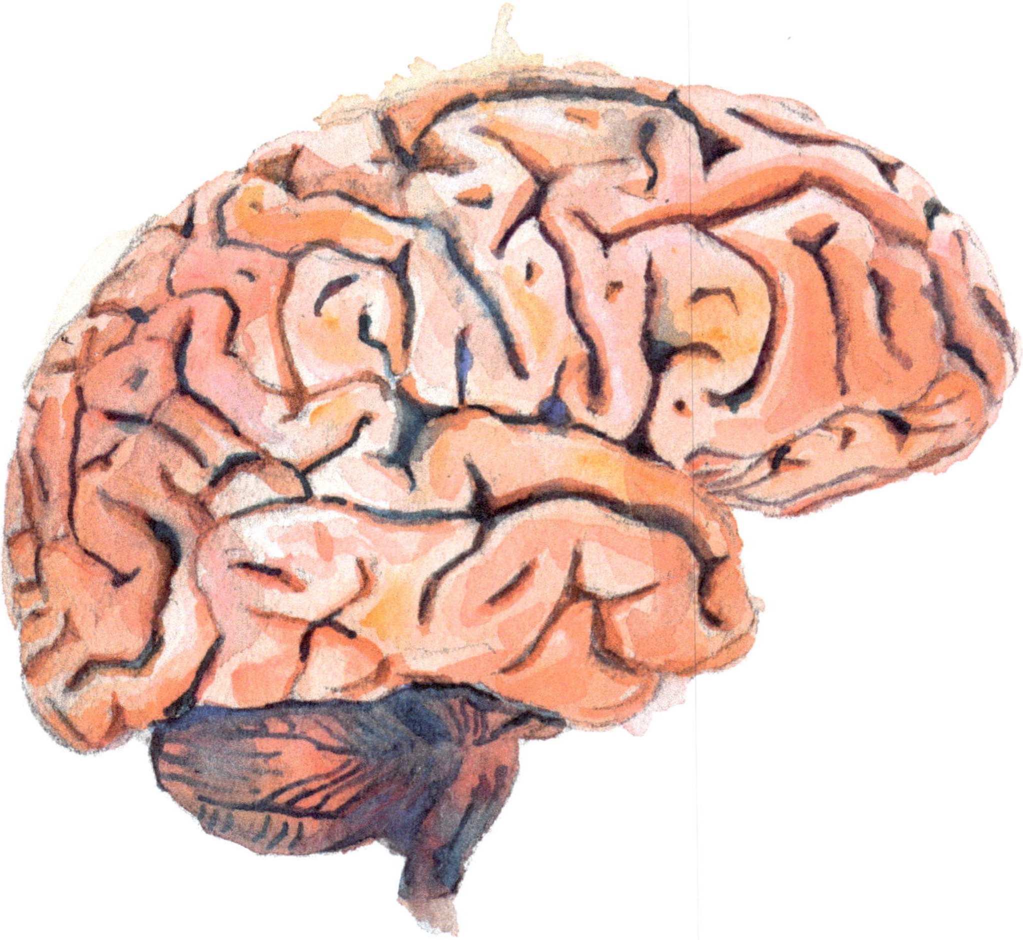

Sagittal Brain
8x10 Watercolor
2015

chapter four

SOME ORGANS

"As man has a pool of blood in which the lungs rise and fall in breathing, so the body of the earth has its ocean tide which likewise rises and falls every six hours, as if the world breathed."

-Leonardo Da Vinci

The Liver
8x10 Watercolor
2016

LIVER, OH LIVER

Liver, liver, why do I treat you so bad?
I think because I can't see when you're sad.
I know I won't hear a complaint 'til too late.
In the meantime, my other needs seem too great.
And also, let's admit, you do ask for much,
So many tasties you say I can't touch.
I'd treat you better if you weren't so damned picky;
And if those liver lobules weren't so persnickety.
Like why are hepatocytes so desperate for salad?
Roasted red meat is so much less pallid!
And who wants just water all night and all day?
A drink is well-earned late on a Friday.
Yes, it's Friday, as I write this to you
And in my hand? It's a marg (or two).
Liver, oh liver, it's not that I don't care...
Next week I'll do better, really I swear.
(Or maybe perhaps the week after that.
Cause I think there's a wine tasting I want be at.)

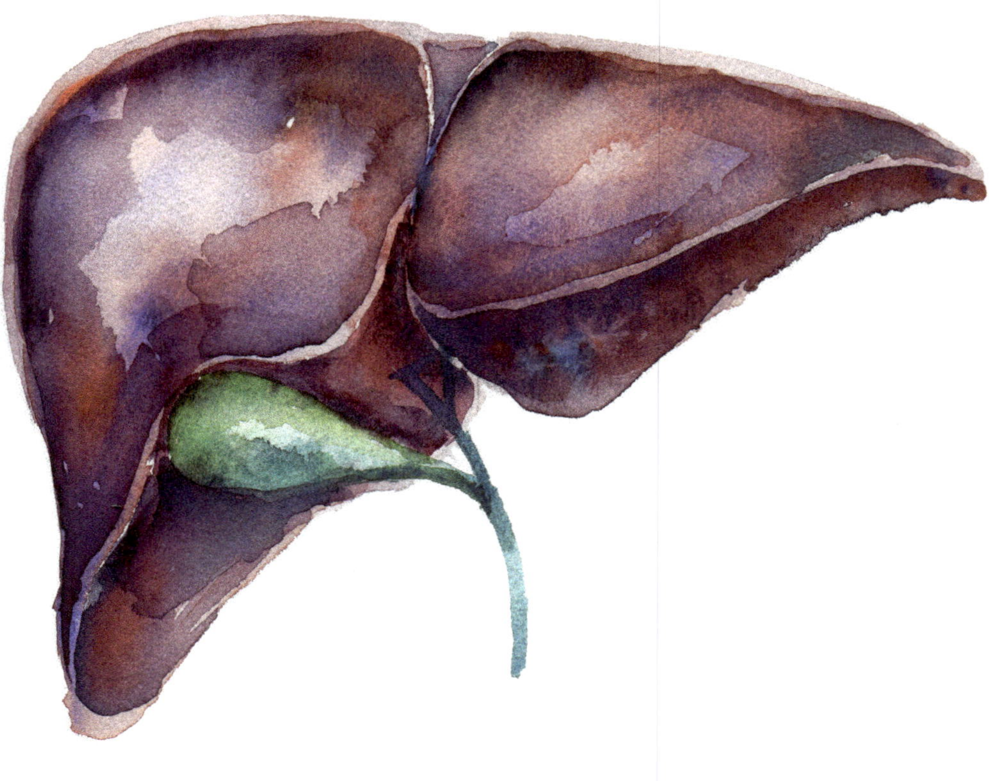

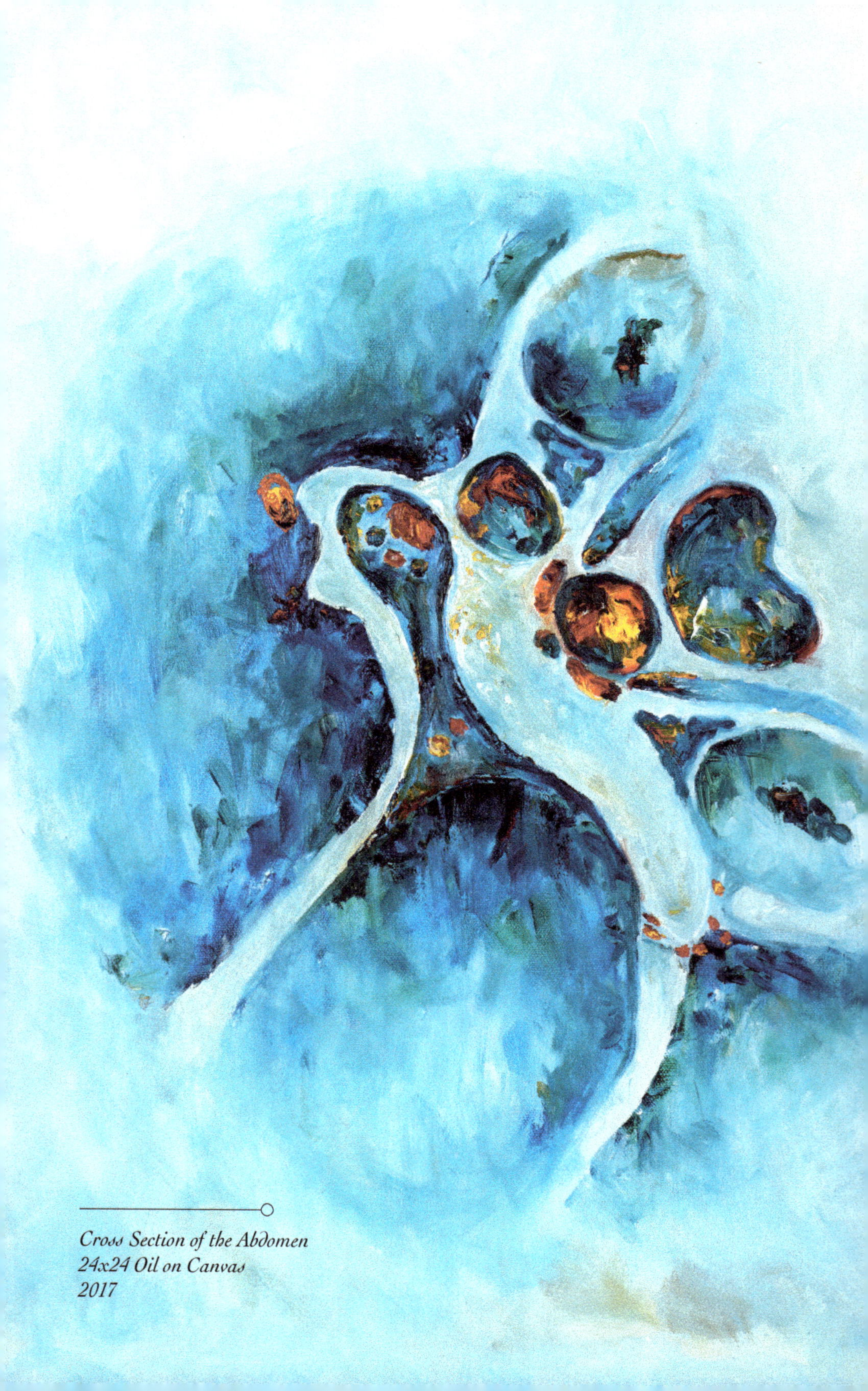

Cross Section of the Abdomen
24x24 Oil on Canvas
2017

STOMACH ACHE

Doctor! Doctor! Alert! Alert!
Please help me, my stomach hurts!
Perhaps I'm menstruating a little early?
It can't be a kidney infection, surely?
Do you think I am lactose intolerant?
(Is that gene even dominant?)
Gastritis seems too general a term…
I traveled recently; do I have worms?
This cramping has just reminded me
That IBS runs in my family!
Or wait, oh no, I bet it's Crohn's
Or my gallbladder has made some stones?
The food I had last night was iffy.
And an ulcer is possible, you must agree!
I've heard complaints of a stomach flu.
Wait, is that a hernia, poking through?
I fell skiing, is my spleen punctured?
Maybe my appendix ruptured!
Or maybe—TOOT!—Oh, excuse that rumble!
I guess it was just a big gas bubble!

SKIN

I am the epidermis,
Thin and tough
I protect the innards
Through good times and rough.
I grow new skin cells
When the old ones slough
I am the epidermis,
Thin and tough.

I am the dermis,
Crowded and thick.
I have nerves and vessels
And sweat glands so slick.
I'm rife with proteins
That keep me elastic.
I am the dermis,
Crowded and thick.

I am the hypodermis,
Heavy and warm
I'm filled with fat
That'll cushion a storm.
I store some energy
That can later transform.
I am the hypodermis,
Heavy and warm.

Skin Histology
9x12 Watercolor
2019

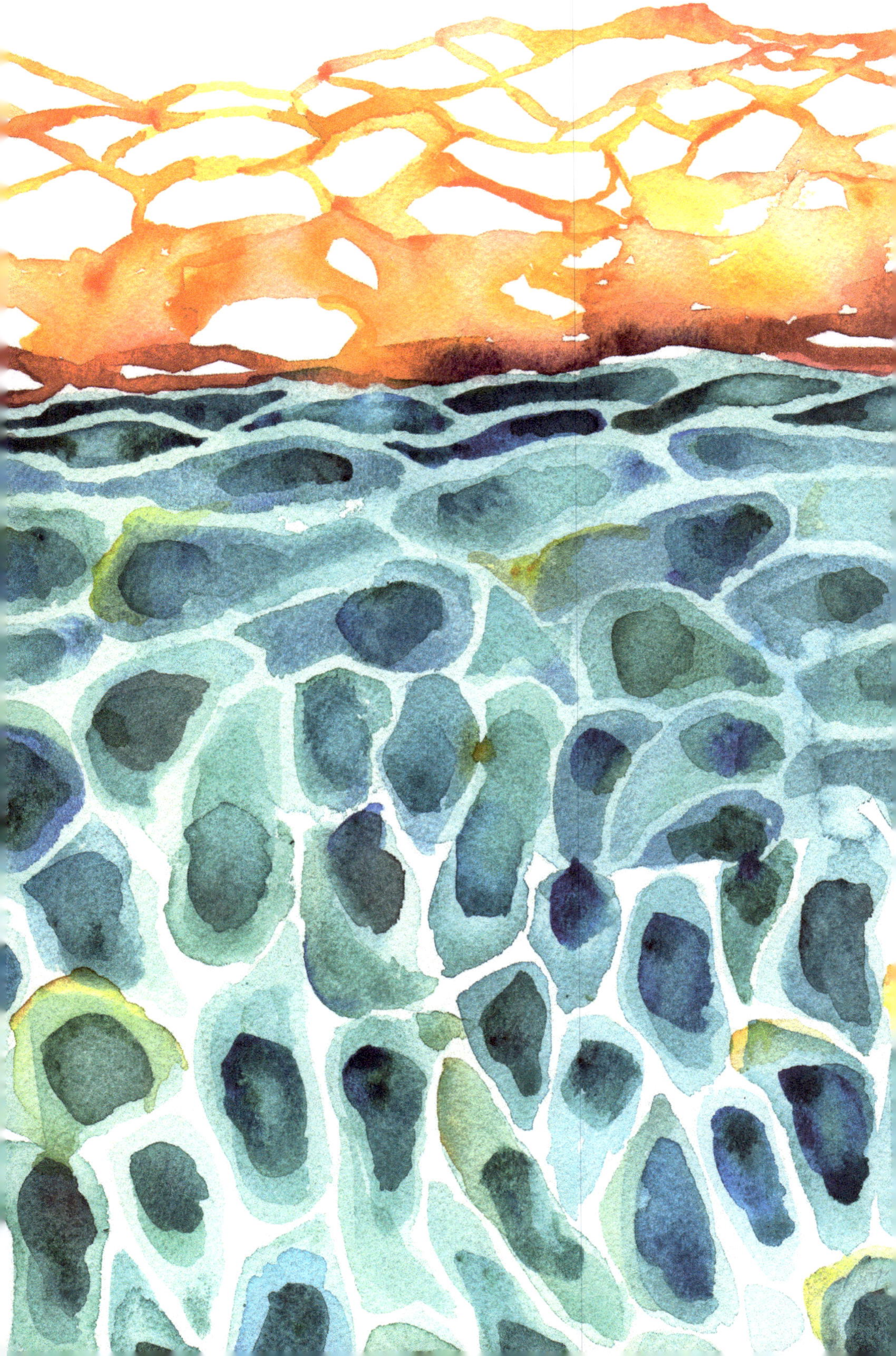

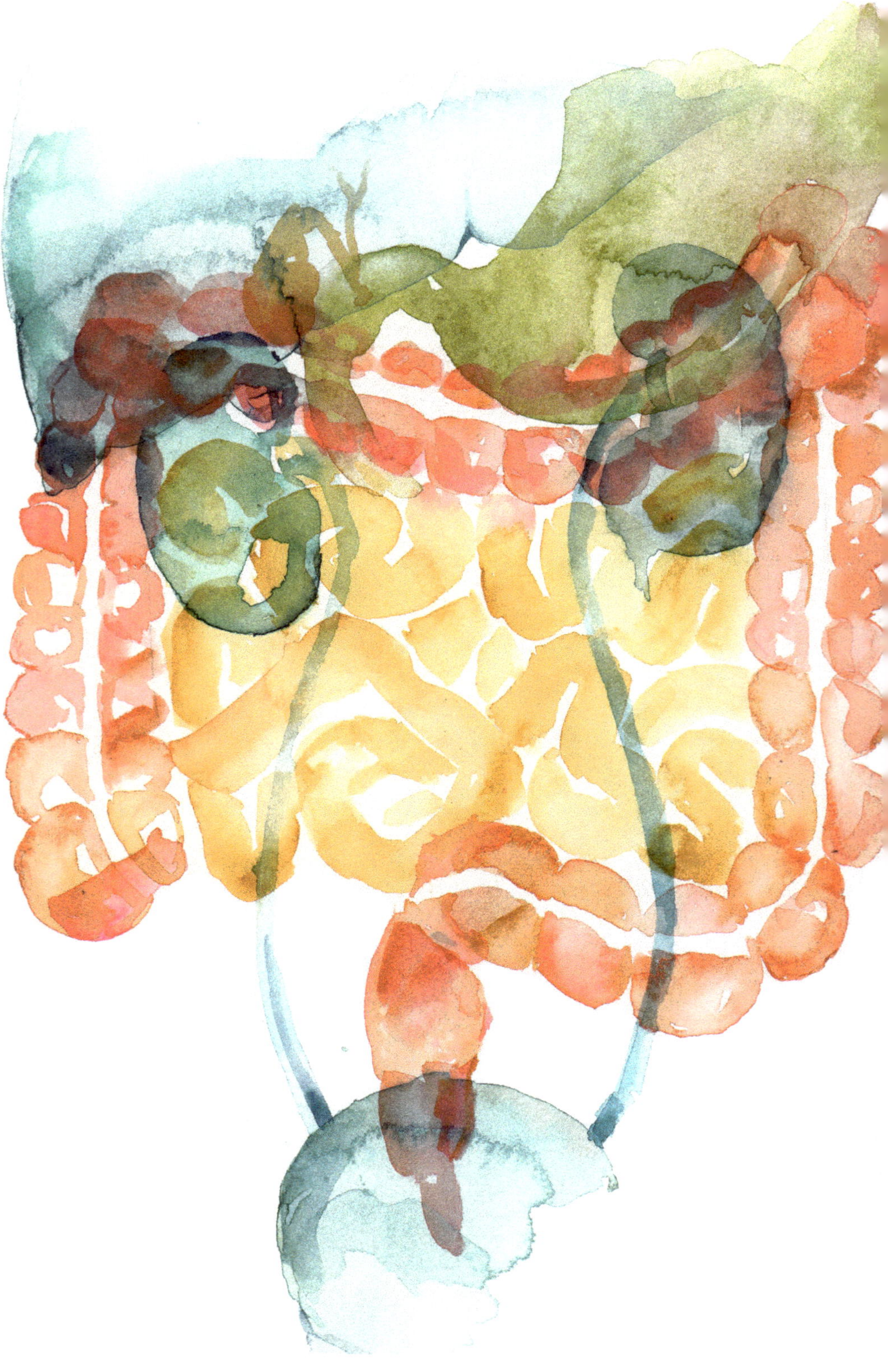

PLUMBING I

Wee pipes, lean pipes, mighty pipes, flighty pipes
All contribute to our indoor plumbing.
A system of filters, muscles and tubes
That keeps that warm, wet urine coming.

Itty tubies, bitty tubies found within the kidney
Filter water and waste from blood.
Nutrients can then be reabsorbed
Before eventually secreting a flood.

To tunnels so long, tunnels so strong,
Urine gets pushed along their ducts.
(But watch out for that splashback curse
Of vesicoureteral reflux.)

A rising tide, the urine bides,
Getting comfy at the Bladder Inn.
'Til the detrusor contracts, the sphincters relax
And micturition can begin.

The slide that's last is rather fast
Pushing out pee with clear perfection
Well, not quite perfect, given the prevalence
Of urinary tract infections.

This team of pipes should get more hype
As they take care of many situations.
Like blood volume, pH and pressure
And all your basic osmoregulation.

GI/GU System
16x20 Watercolor
2023

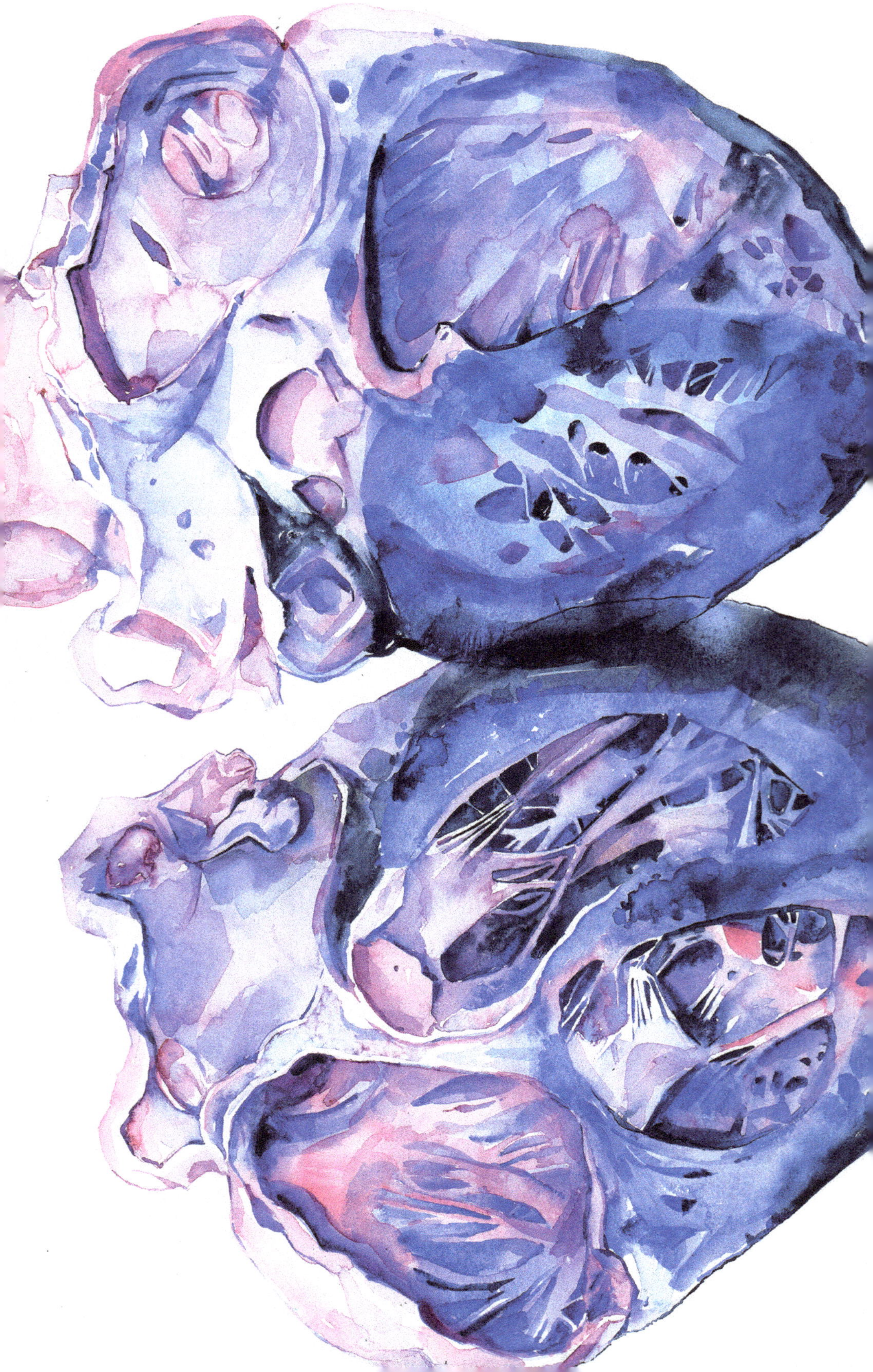

CHORDAE TENDINEAE

I seek to unearth places of beauty inside;
Deep in the heart such a region resides.

A pillowy parachute rippling with grace,
Flowing in time with the heart's pumping pace.

With silky white strings, each chordae tendineae
Prevent the valve flaps from floating away.

By forming a web tethered taught to a mound
Of papillary muscle, tall and proud.

Imagine those cords as they sway and they slide
With the ebb and flow of a crimson tide.

Such delicate ropes, but they hide in their length
A surfeit of endurance and unending strength.

For these exquisite strands manage the feat
Of holding on tight for a lifetime of beats.

My Heart is Blue
22x30 Watercolor
2022

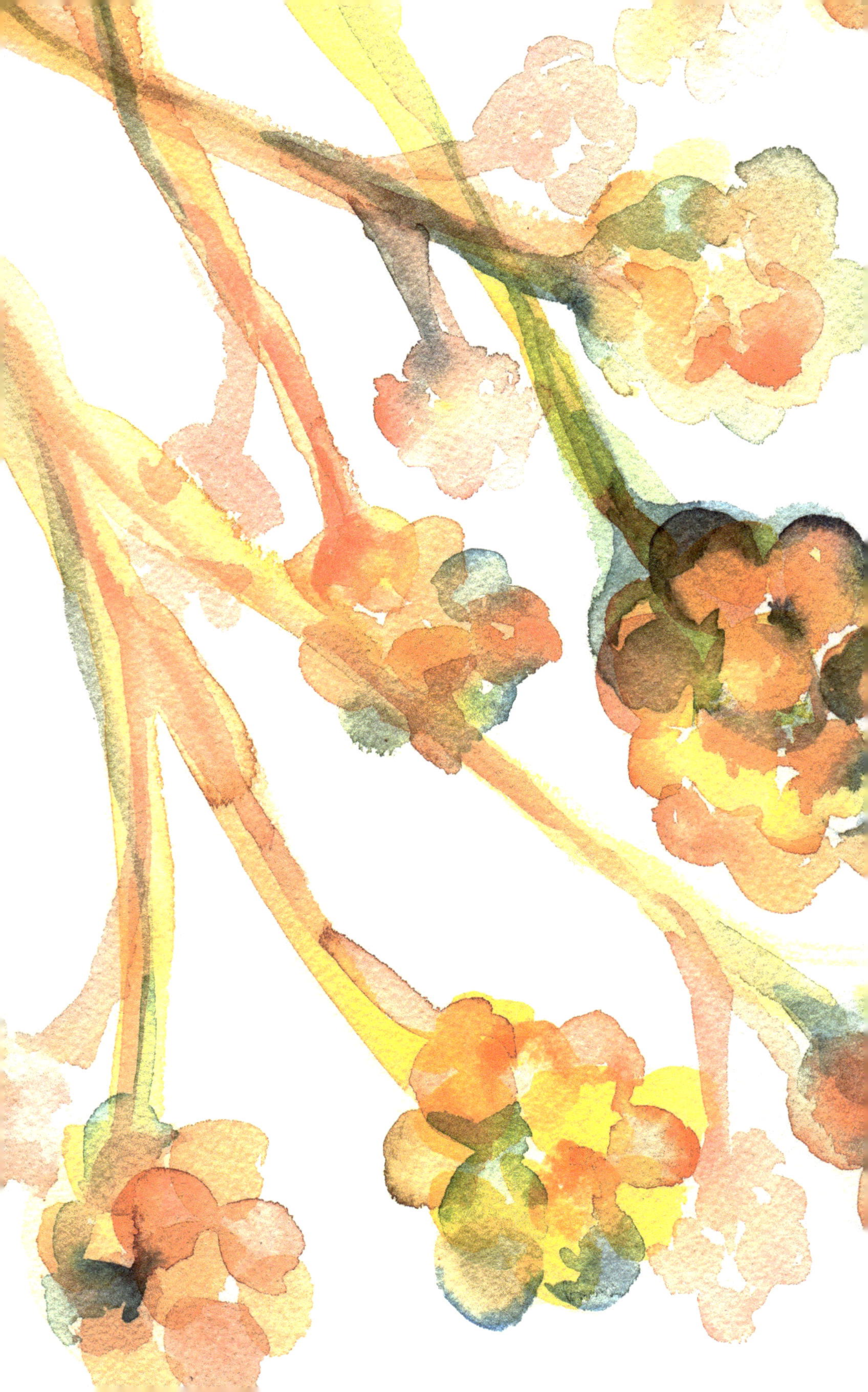

ALVEOLI

Air flows in the mouth and nose
While we wait.
Air gushes through the trachea hose
While we wait.

Through two bronchi the air now flees
While we bide.
It travels along the bronchial tree
While we bide.

Now it reaches the bronchioles
While we hold.
And now it's nearing our tiny holes
While we hold...

And WHOOSH!

Out it goes.

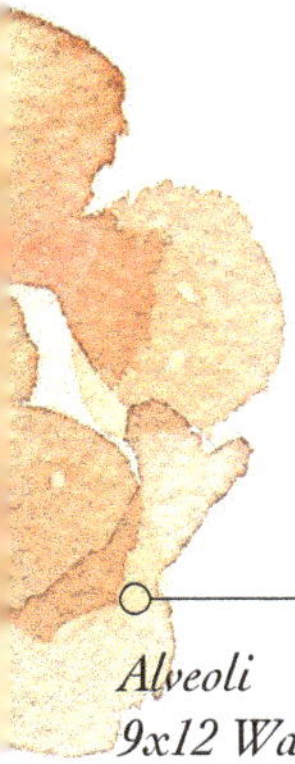

Alveoli
9x12 Watercolor
2016

MIC DROP

I, the brain, am at the top, and better than all you rot
Because if I'm not here, none of you can even function.
I'm basically magic the way I use e-signals to plot
Ways to not let y'all physiologically malfunction.
*Mic drop

I, the heart, I am the start and end of this operation,
Why else would my name imply the very essence of a thing?
For without me and my pulsating cellular population,
All the bloody junk you need no one would ever, ever bring.
*Mic drop

We, the lungs, we know we're apex amongst all of you basics.
See, from the air out there we suck in a breezy bolus of vitality,
Stop that and you'll be a desert lacking an oxygenated oasis
Plus, our calm breath brings crazy brain back to some normality.
*Mic drop

I, the appendix, I'm not really sure if I can compete.
I'm actually not really sure what I'm here for or what I even do.
But I hope you guys still treat me really nice and sweet.
*OR I'LL LOSE MY MIND AND EXPLODE AND TRY TO
KILL ALL OF YOU!*
*Mic drop

Appendicitis
16x22 Pen and Watercolor
2024

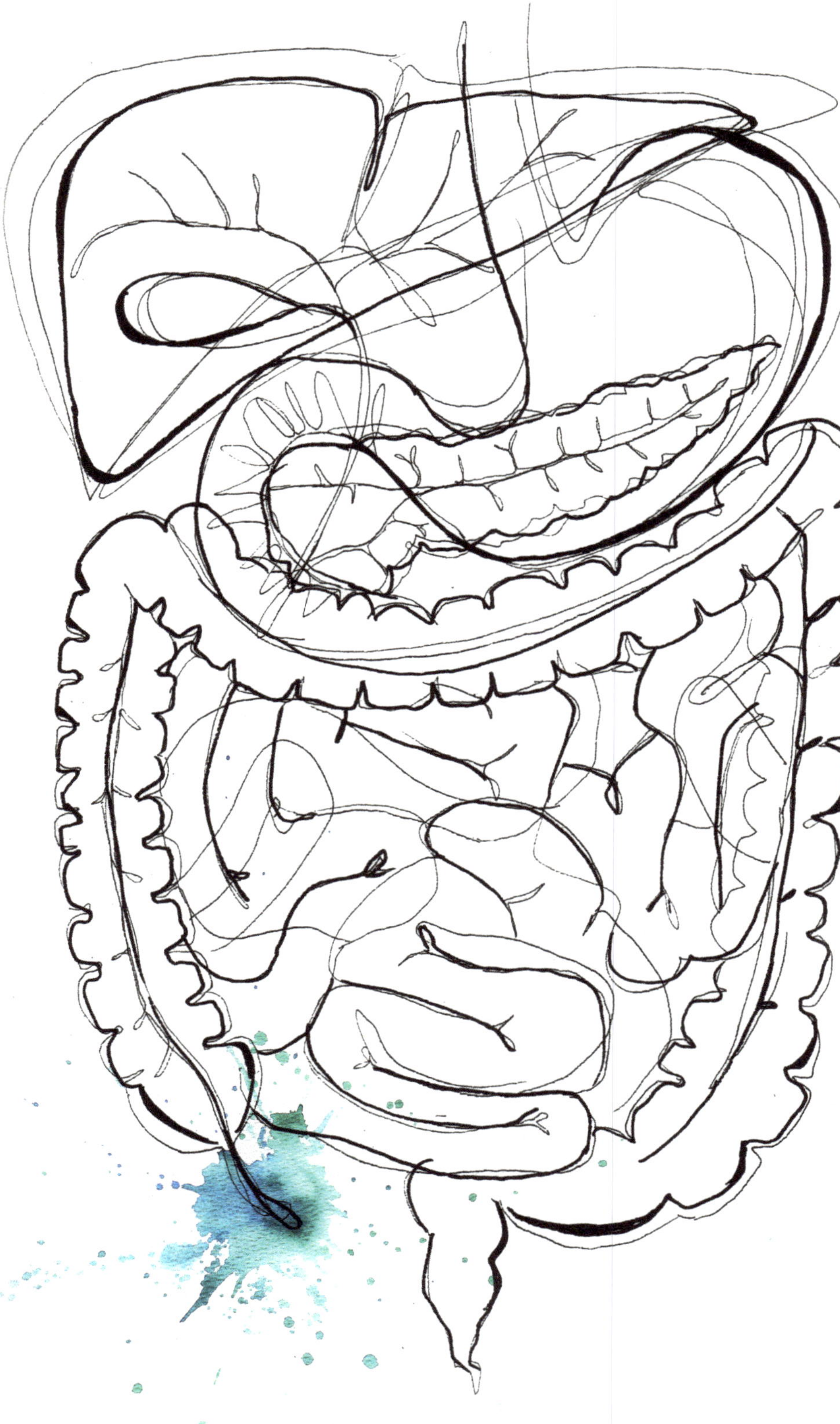

THE RACE

In the right atrium my race begins,
Then through the trapdoor on the floor.
I stop to rest but to my chagrin
The right ventricle shows me the door.

I run to the lungs to get oxygenated,
Then it's back to the left side of the heart.
It's easier now since I'm sated,
So through atrium and ventricle I dart.

The aorta now flies me up and out
But right away I have to split up
In order to deliver oxygen about
The body, from bottom to top

At the capillaries I make the exchange,
Trading the blue, tired blood for my red
Suddenly I feel so tired and strange,
If it weren't for these vein valves I'd be dead!

I pant and I chug and then see as I moan
The finish line—the heart—I'm almost in it!
Inferior vena cava, please bring me home...
Did that really all just take a minute?

Bold Heart
8x10 Watercolor
2021

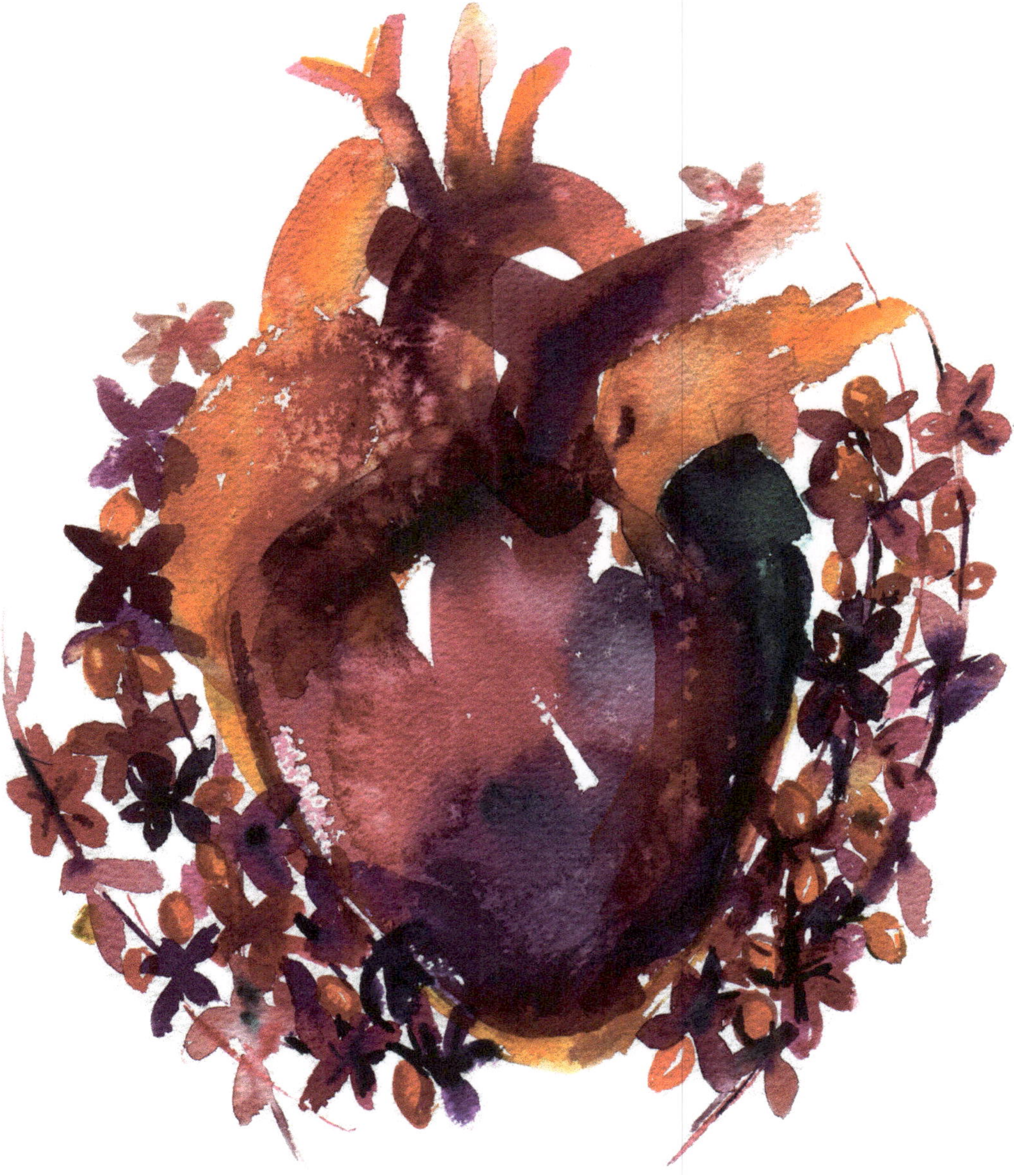

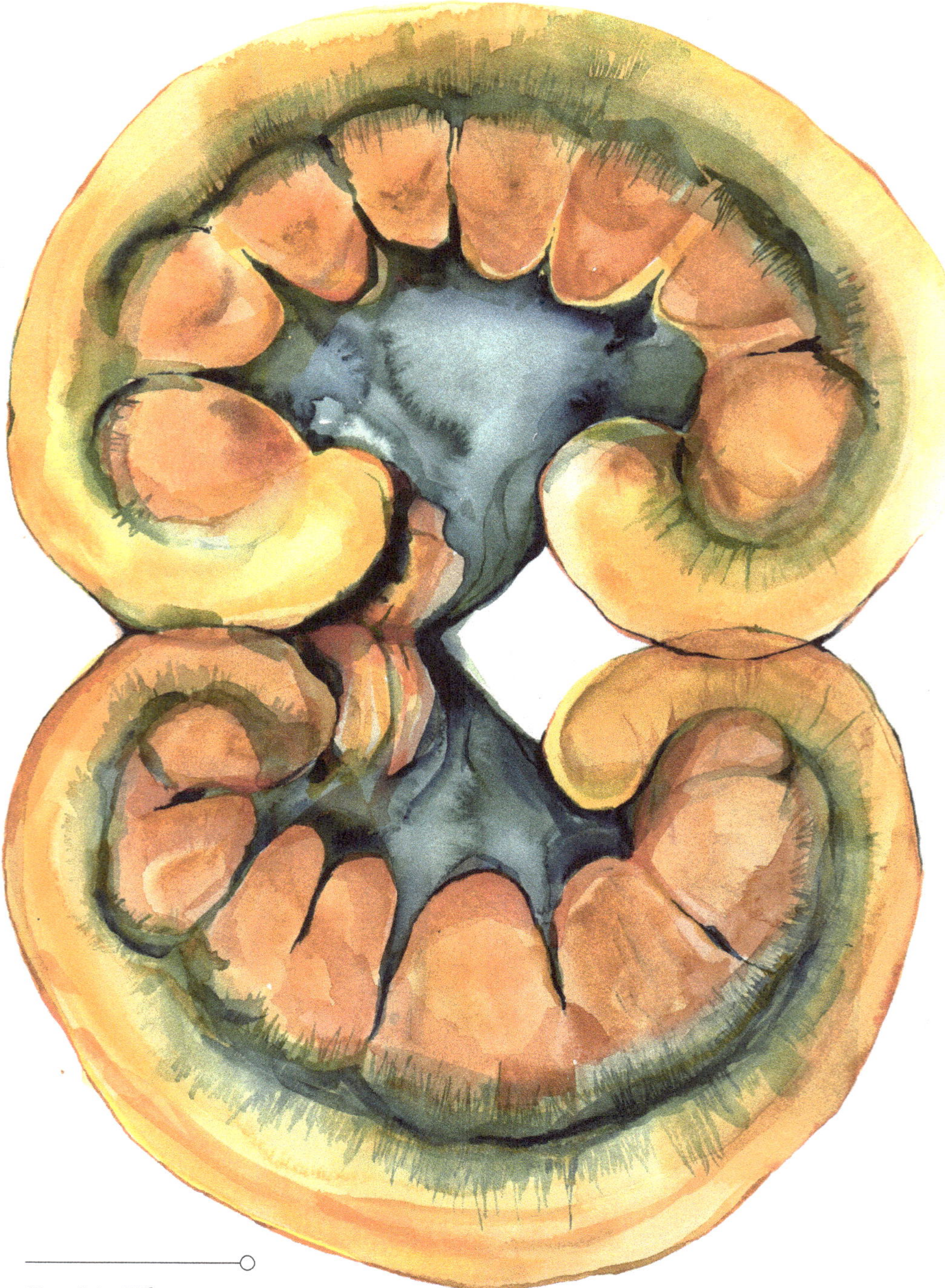

Exquisite Kidney
18x22 Watercolor
2021

RENAL PYRAMIDS

Within the kidney is a curious soul,
A bundle of tissue dubbed the renal pyramid.
Stabilizing water and salt is its goal,
And making the blood all good again.

Yes, blood! Did you know it gets bad?
From acid and toxins and imbalanced water.
But once it flows through the pyramid's pad,
It is no longer a maroon marauder.

How is this so? How does it begin?
How does a triangular mass fix the mess?
By the loops and twirls of vessels within,
Nephron rivers that mend the duress.

First the blood reaches a twisted old knot,
Referred to as the glomerulus.
Pressure gradients force out swill in this spot,
Anything that might be nefarious.

Into a tubule these dregs flow deftly,
And then they embark on a ride
Down and up the steep Loop of Henle
Where they get one last chance to survive.

For the walls here permit reabsorption
Of sodium and water, too.
The concentration gradient decides the portion
Of substances allowed back through.

Eventually waste is all that remains,
And as urine it tinkles au revoir.
Now a perfect balance your body sustains,
Thanks to renal pyramids; I am in awe.

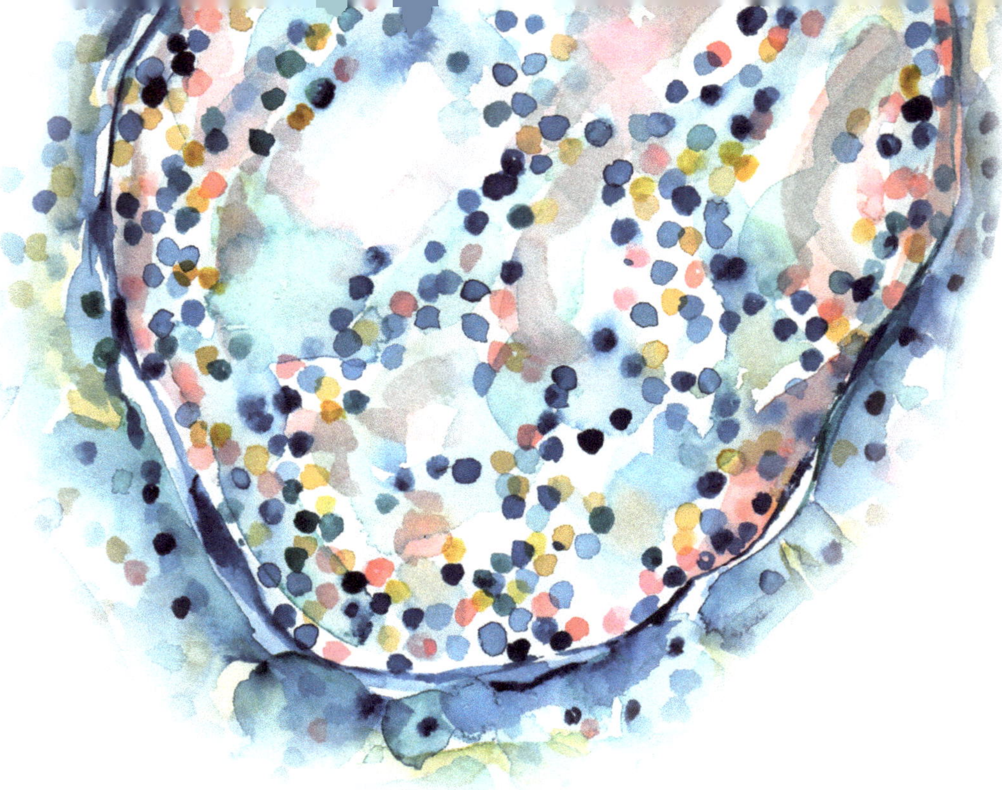

ISLET OF LANGERHANS

Welcome to the pancreas!
You'll soon be thanking us
For this trip inside its fold.

No, you're not in danger, son!
That's just an islet of Langerhans,
To that cluster of cells, let's go!

There's a surge now, watch out!
No, no, don't shout,
It's just a glucagon and insulin wave.

Did that flood almost drown you?
Well now, don't frown, you.
Those hormones keep diabetes away.

Islet of Langerhans
8x10 Watercolor
2021

GLOMERULUS

Squirmy, wormy cluster.
Ew, I can barely muster
Any respect for that
Squishy, vessely vat.
But respect it does demand
For the fact that it can
Filter out the the shit
That doesn't keep me fit.
So buh-bye water and waste,
Leave my body with haste.
Make room for the good stuff,
Within this capillary tuft.
Like little bits of protein,
And things that make blood clean.
You know, it would be a challenge
To keep my fluids in balance,
If it weren't for glomerulus,
A sieve oh-so-scrupulous.

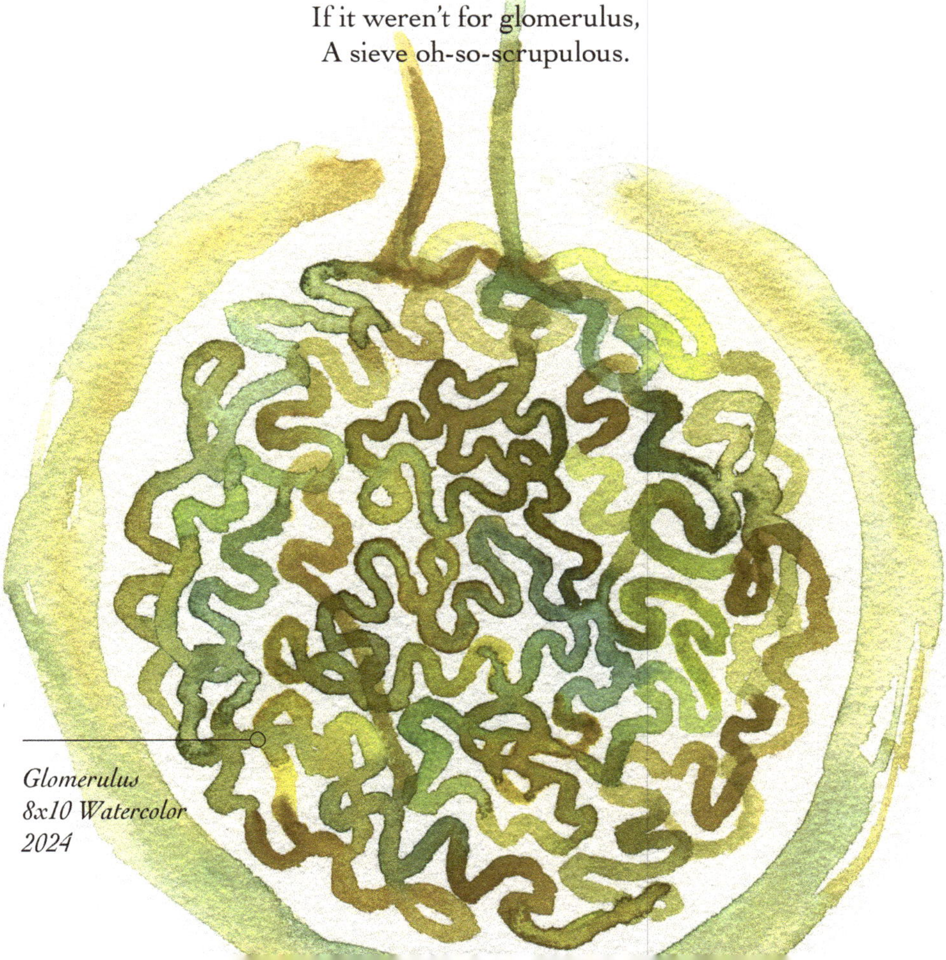

Glomerulus
8x10 Watercolor
2024

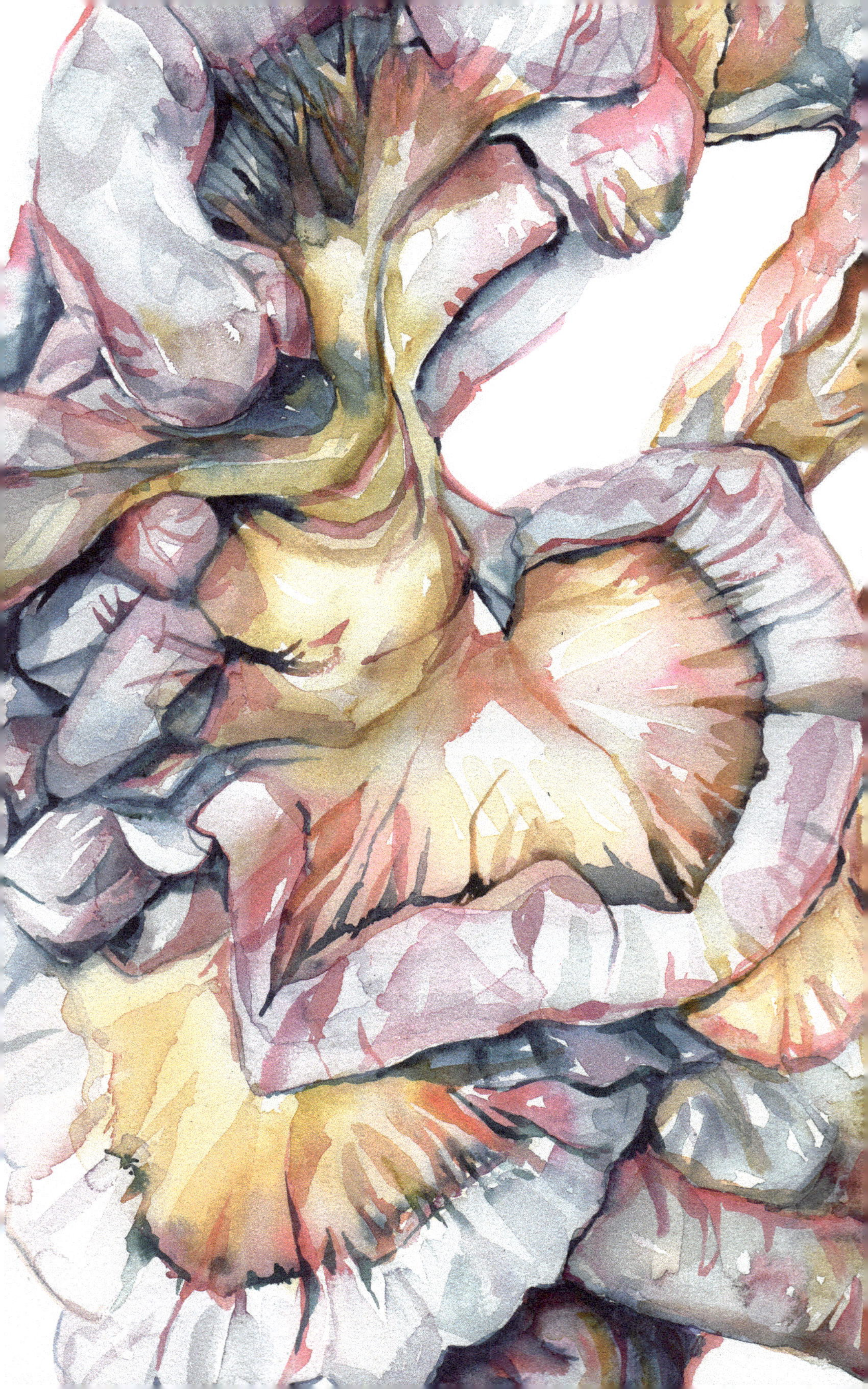

MESENTERY, MESENTERY

Mesentery, mesentery
Without you I'd be so sedentary
Thanks for all your stored energy.
As you keep in place my intestinaries.
I just wish you didn't look so unpleasantary.

Omentum, Omentum
While you give immune guys momentum,
We all took a referendum
And decided you're name is dumb
Since you're just fat spread over the tum-tum.

Peritoneum, Peritoneum.
(Not to be confused with perineum.)
You're like an abdominal museum.
You give the other two their freedom,
Although they're still a part of your kingdom.

Exquisite Mesentery
16x22 Watercolor
2022

PLUMBING II

Food gets swish-y inside of the squishy
Tubes of the digestive tract.
Let's find a liking for our inner piping
That empties our waste out the back.

The stomach makes chyme and then it's time
For the duodenum to have some fun.
Enzymes are poured, nutrients get stored,
Then the chyme continues its run.

To the jejunum and ileum, both with a trillion
Microvilli which ceaselessly absorb
Water and nourishment, then block with discouragement
The waste that it cannot store.

Perhaps it's cruel, but we now call it stool
When the leftovers enter the colon.
Up, over and down, the stool goes around
Traveling along in slow motion.

Now you may be aware that the colon needs care.
Sudden changes will stop it from going.
Give it fiber and liquid, or it'll be restricted.
Though if you squat, things'll get rolling.

After it finishes its route and the stool comes out
Through the rectum and a couple of sphincters,
You must give it a look, like it's your favorite book,
Because stool is your health predictor.

Colonoscopy
8x10 Watercolor
2021

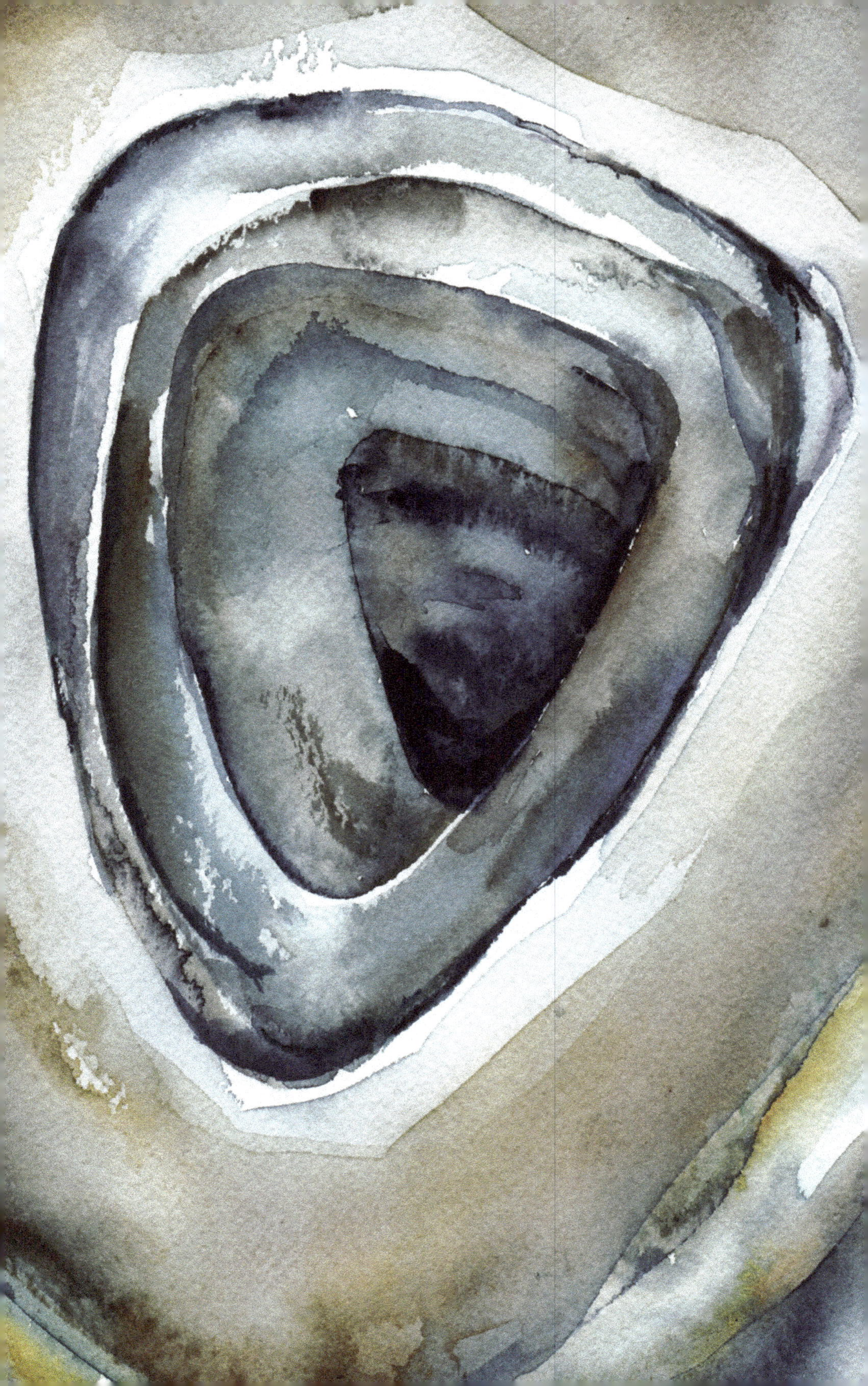

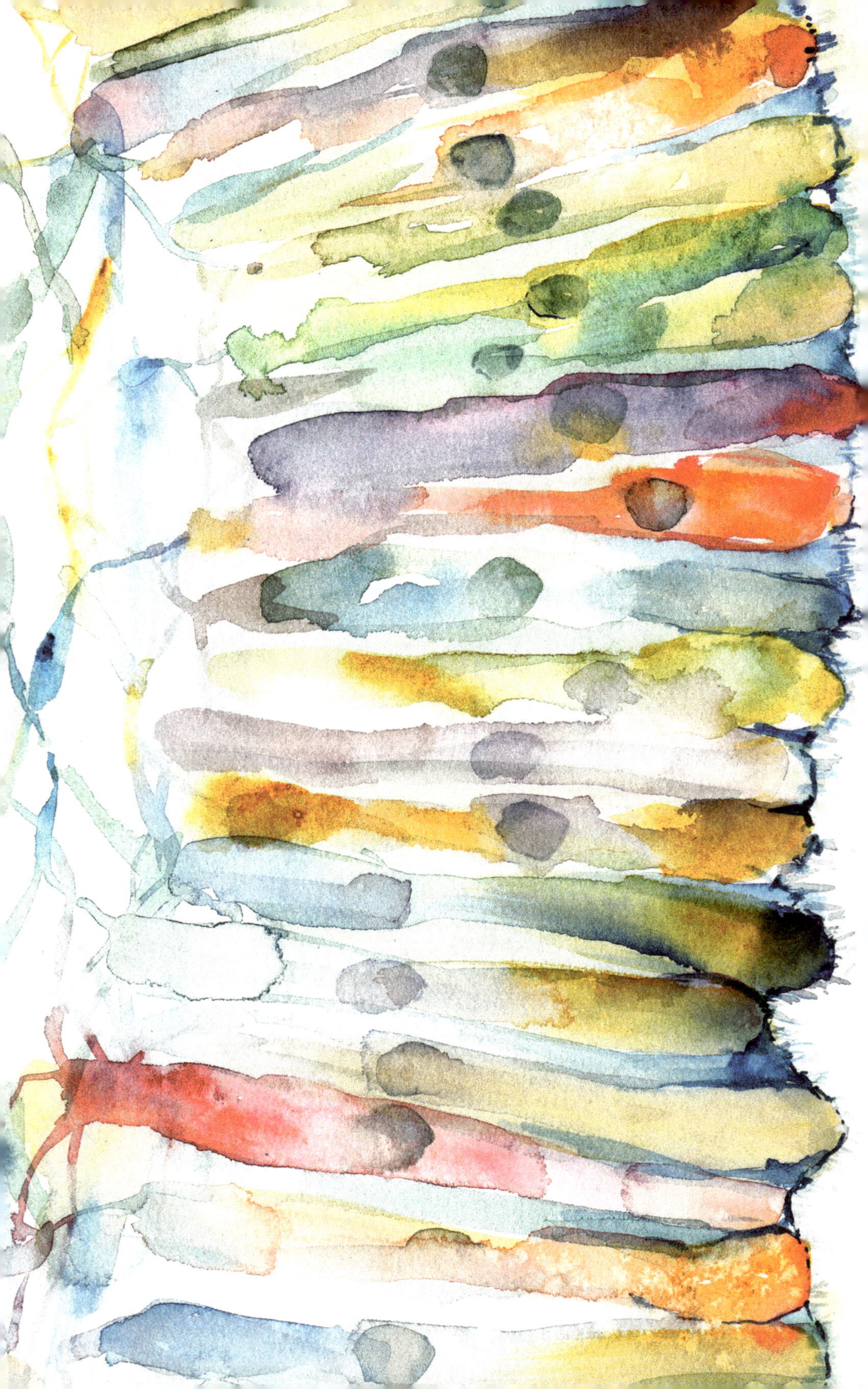

MICROVILLI

Sure, some nutrients soak in
As food passes your chin
And slides down past your craw.

But "Not enough!" Body will cry
Good thing for microvilli,
Each one like a miniscule straw.

In just one millimeter of intestine
200 million are destined
To be a vitamin and nutrient port

They make gut cells so vast
That were the guts to lie flat
They'd be the size of a tennis court.

Microvilli
9x12 Watercolor
2019

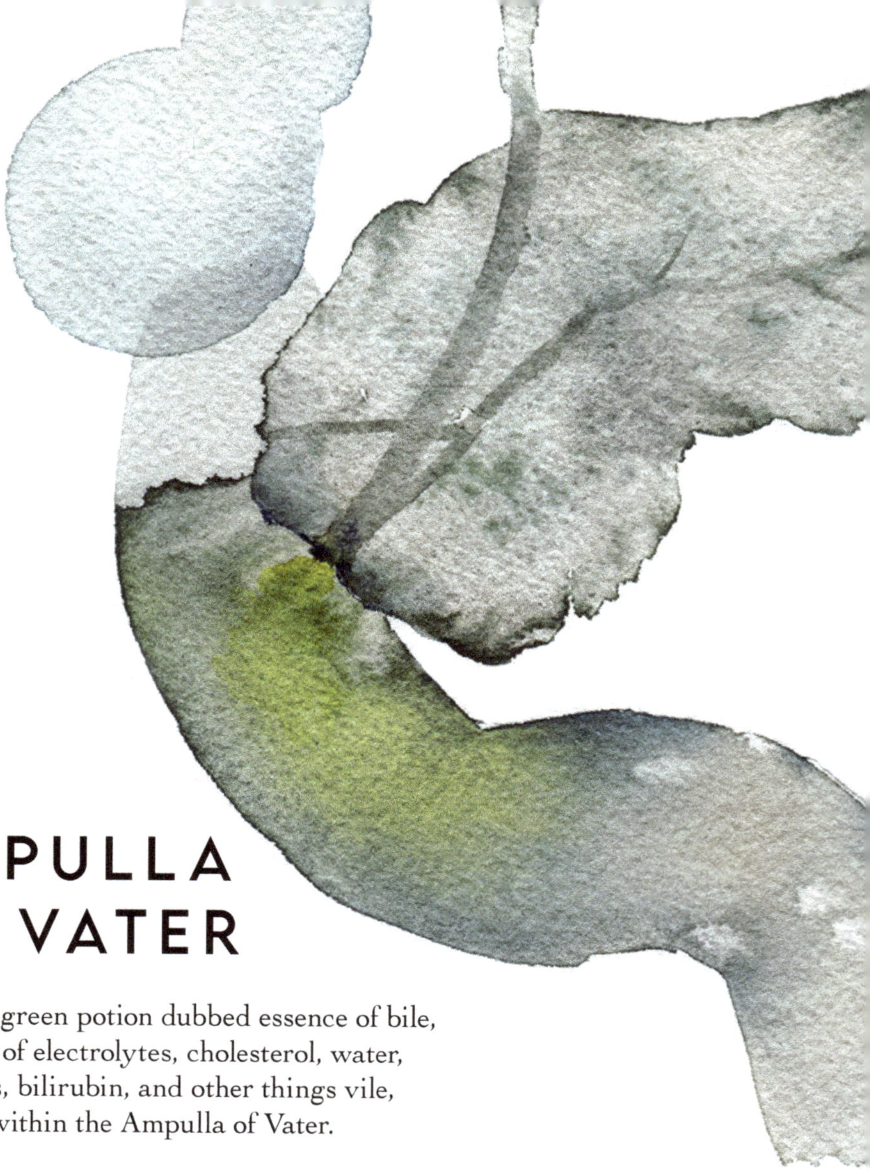

AMPULLA OF VATER

A yellow-green potion dubbed essence of bile,
Made up of electrolytes, cholesterol, water,
Bile acids, bilirubin, and other things vile,
Gurgles within the Ampulla of Vater.

From the liver these additives were plucked,
Then flowed through some torpid canals.
They land within the Common Bile Duct,
Where the Cystic and Hepatic pipes corralled.

But before the drink is ready to brine
It requires a mysterious mixer.
From the pancreatic duct some digestive enzymes
Will be added to the final elixir.

Within the ampulla, the potion's amassed
Chartreuse and viscous, it's ready at last.

Ampulla of Vater
8x10 Watercolor
2023

chapter five

SPECIAL SENSES

"The senses are of the earth, the reason stands apart from them in contemplation."

-Leonardo Da Vinci

I CHOOSE THE LIGHT

Our senses compile the surrounding world.
Sights, sounds and more unceasingly hurled.
But there is a choice in what gets unfurled.
I want to do right.

Entertainment always within reach of my fingers.
Seductively charming, the fun of it lingers.
But it brings a dusk to dreamers and thinkers.
I must ward off that night.

It's daunting to choose in each case and space
To put mental nourishment in front of my face.
But with the hope of a bright, glowing grace,
I embrace the light.

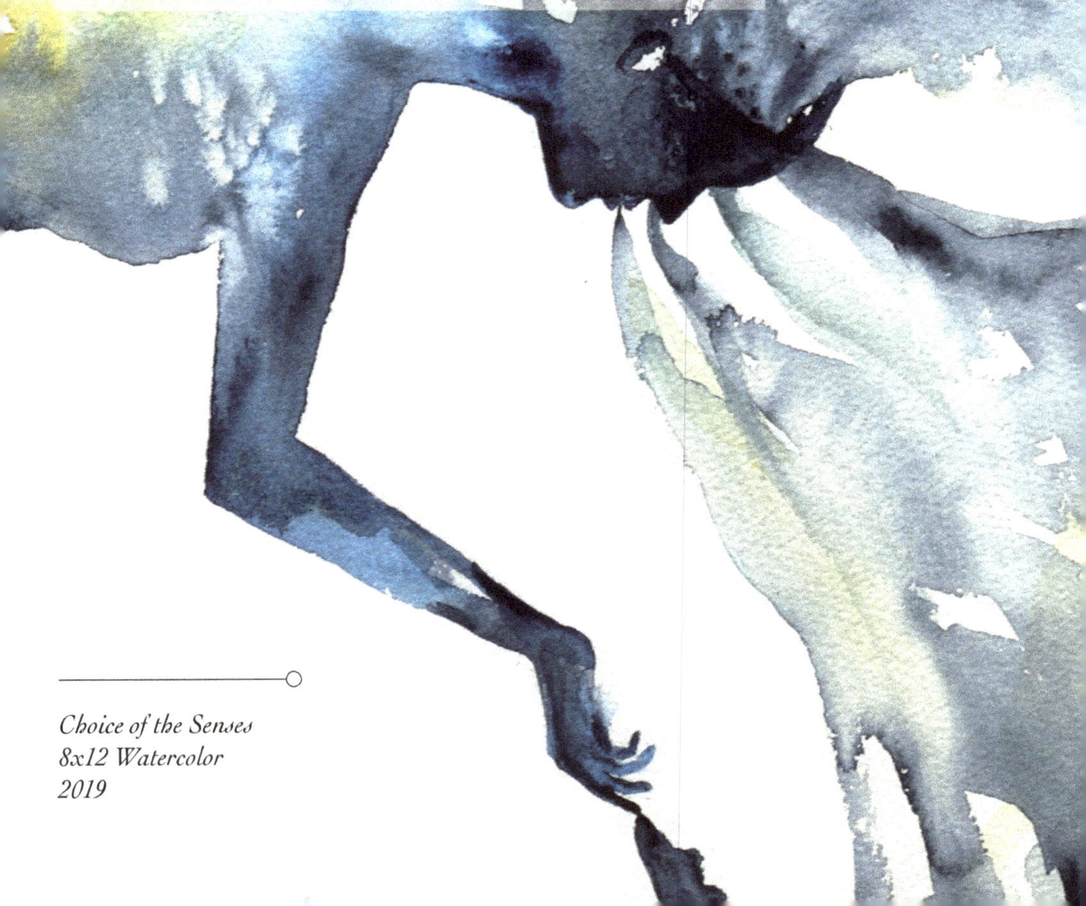

Choice of the Senses
8x12 Watercolor
2019

I FEEL

I feel
I feel my child's hand
        nestled in mine
Touch cells awaken,
        purr with contentment
A warm wind of sunshine
        sweeps through my heart
I feel joy and hope and contentment and life
        and love
All because
I feel.

Touch Horizons: Pacinian Corpuscle
22x30 Watercolor
2018

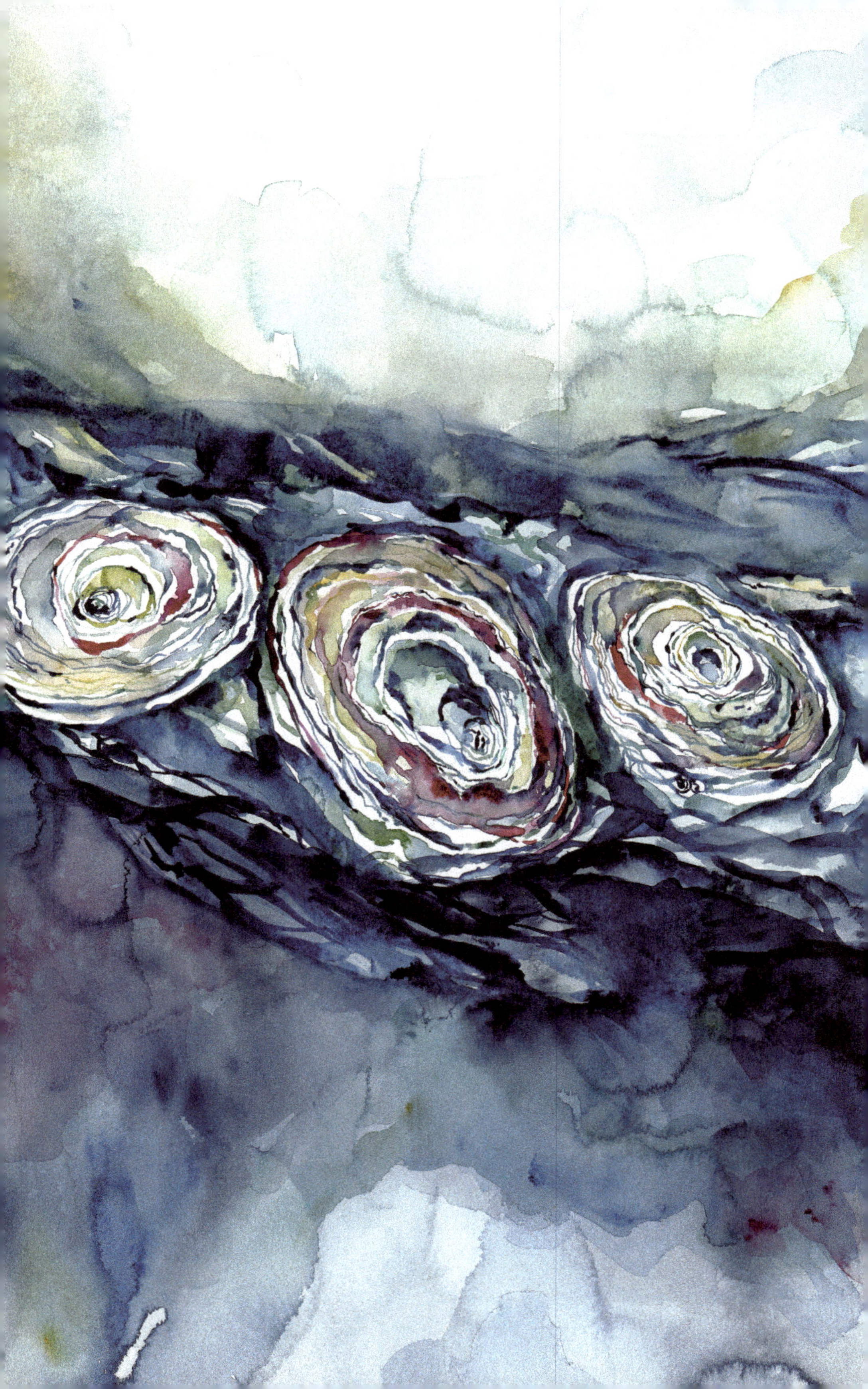

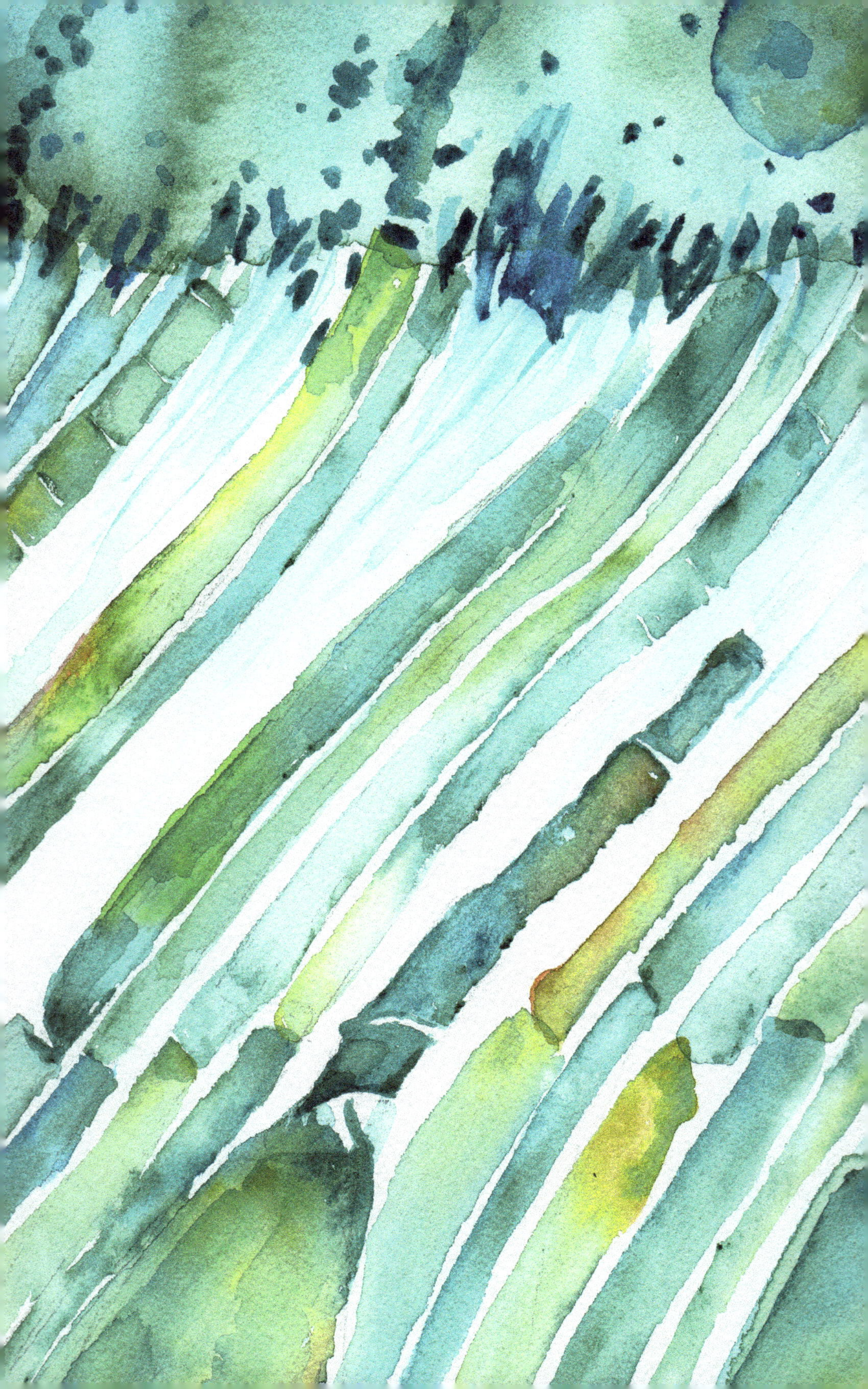

RODS OR CONES

Rods or cones!
Rods or cones!
Two sensory cells
that both want the throne!

Will Cones beat out the rest?
And be labeled the very best?
For only cones see color
And the details expressed!

Or will Rods beat their rival?
With a grayscale revival?
For rods see in low light
And are good for survival!

Cones or rods?
Cones or rods?
Both so cocky; I think I choose...
The bipolar cell squad!

Rods & Cones
9x12 Watercolor
2018

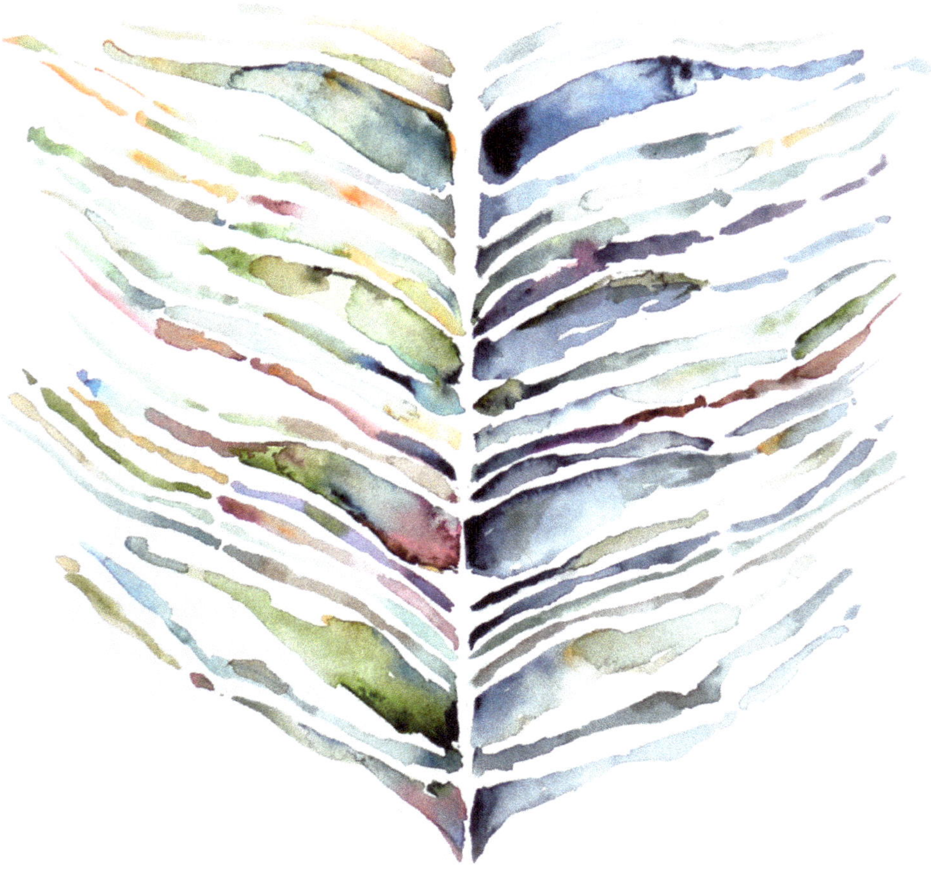

Sight Reflections: Rods and Cones
11x14 Watercolor
2018

I SEE

I see
I see expansive sky
    an impossible blue,
    a cloak of gray,
    an indigo blanket
Rods and cones sizzle as they behold
The everlasting majesty.
And I know
    that I am small
    within this world
Or maybe
    just big enough.
I see.

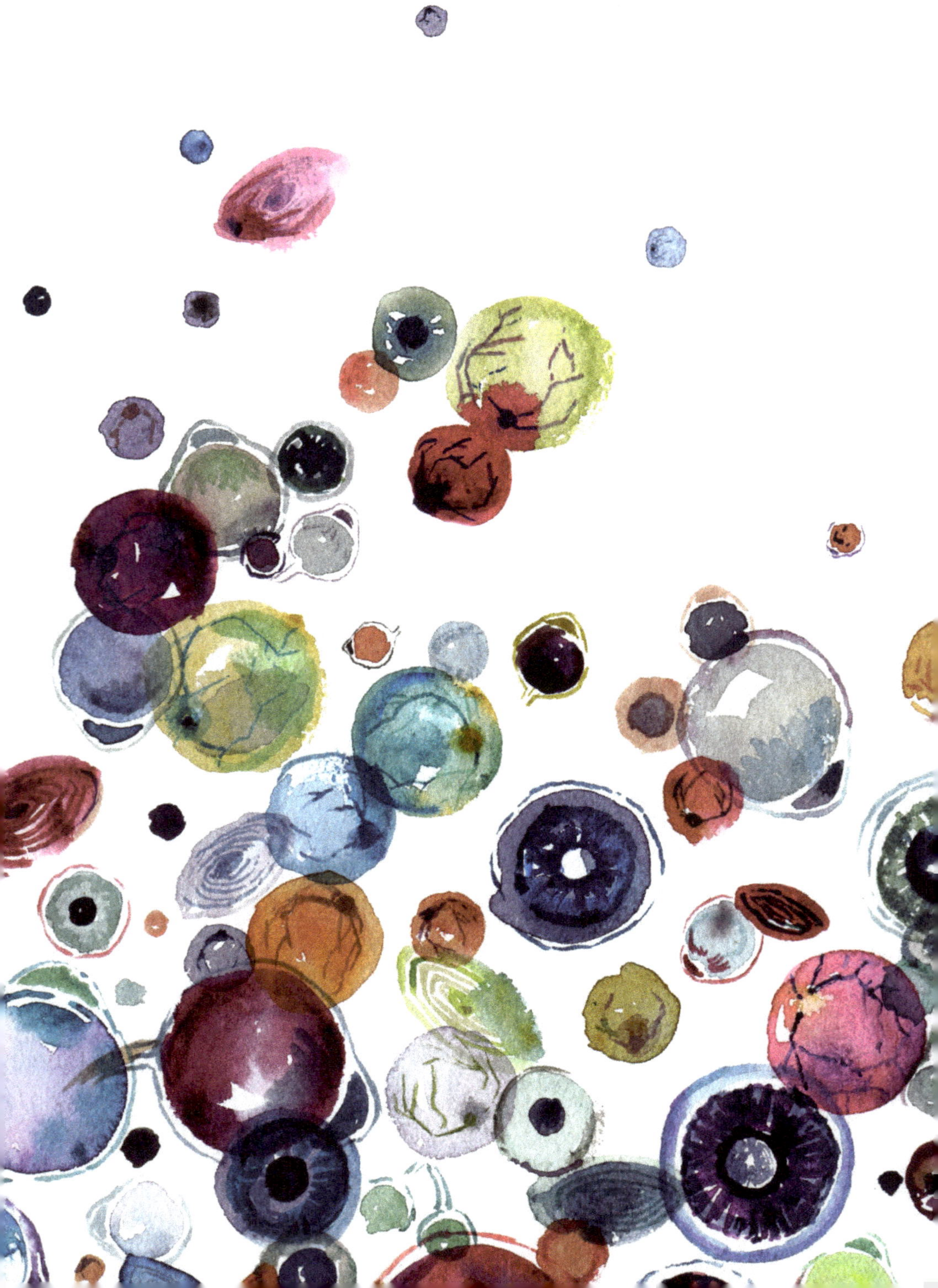

ORA SERRATA

The ora serrata
has a lotta
stress as it circles the eye.

It serves as a bridge
between two things
that don't even like to say hi.

The retina in back
couldn't give a whack
as it's busy transforming the light.

While that ciliary body
is all sorts of dodgy,
stretching the lens day and night.

Eye Things
8x10 Watercolor
2021

I TASTE

I taste
I taste the yeasty cloud of
          my daily bread
Sustenance and joy.
Taste buds sparkle and sing.
But
          is it too good?
          is it too much?
          is it too fake?
A song of guilt rises—
Shhhh
Just taste.

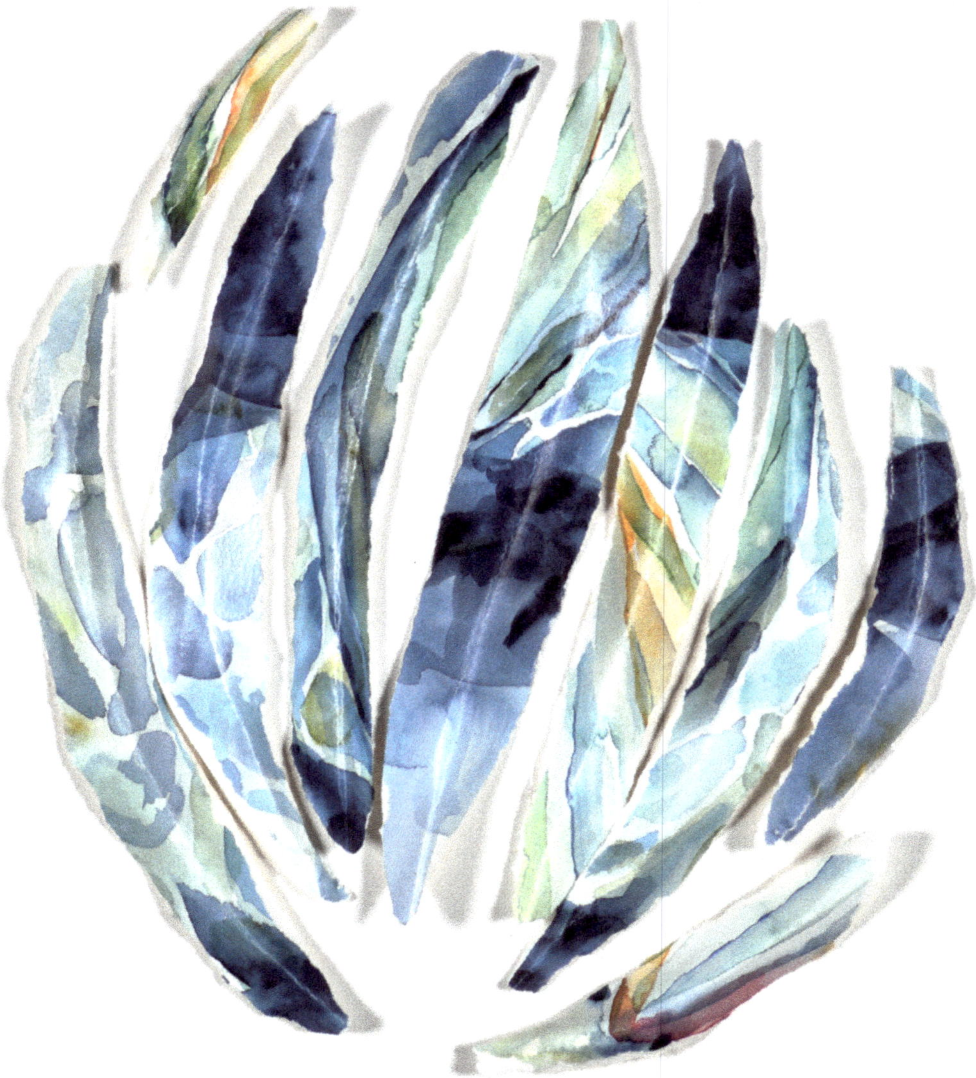

A Taste Bud
16x20 Watercolor, Glue, Varnish
2019

I HEAR

I hear
I hear the whisper of rain
The sound ripples through
A shell in my ear
It patters a promise
Of release and renewal
I am restored
By the rain
I hear

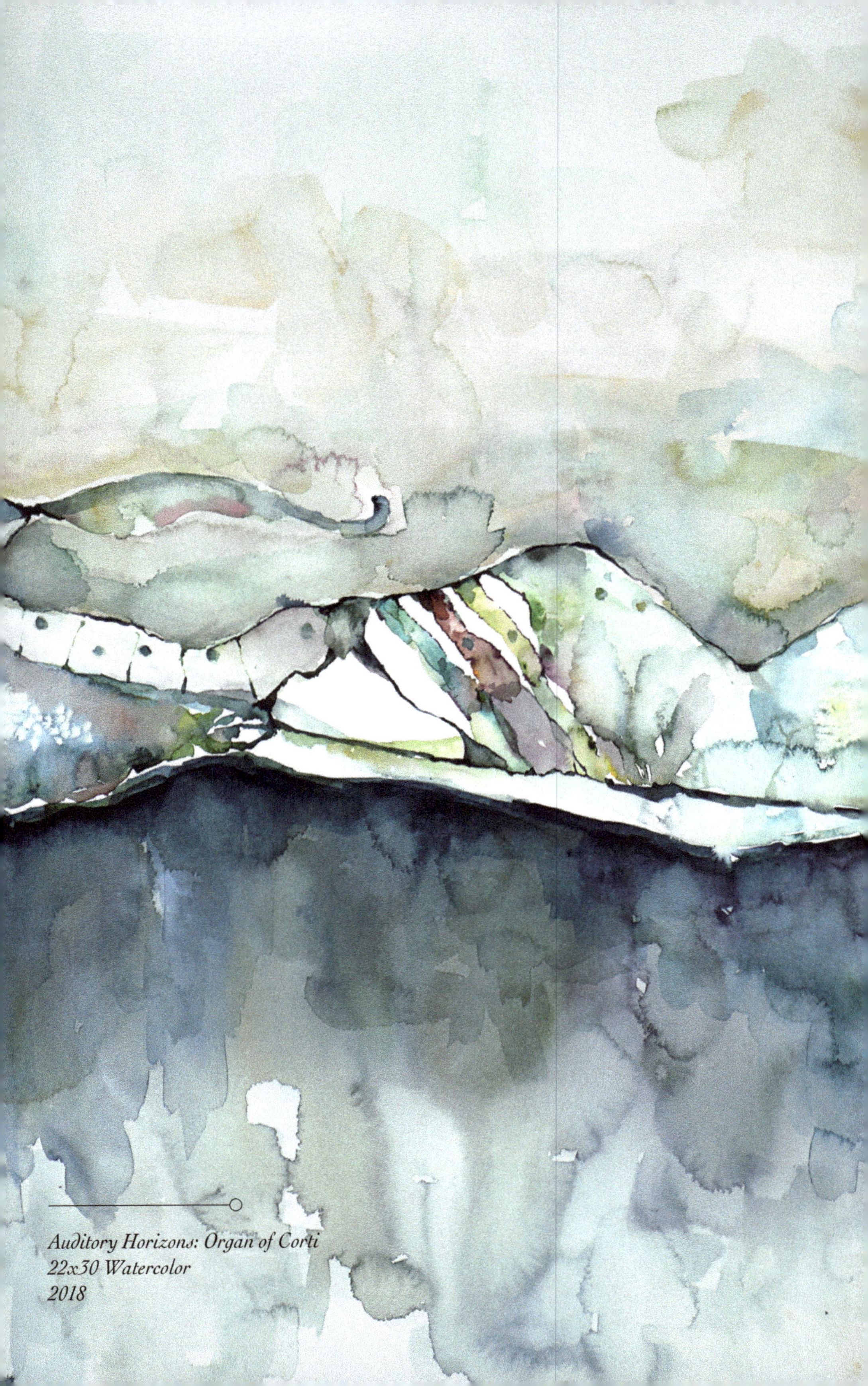

Auditory Horizons: Organ of Corti
22x30 Watercolor
2018

THE COCHLEA

Way deep inside the temporal bone
There's a cave I dub the hearing zone.
A curious sculpture lives in this dell:
The wee cochlea, round like a shell.
An endolymph ocean fills the inside.
Sound makes sense because of its tide,
and the ripples and waves that start to flow,
thanks to vibrations from a little window.
This current gives a tickle, a push,
to special little hairs deep in the mush.
These stereocilia then convert motion
arising from the endolymph ocean
to electrical signals, which then murmur to
thousands of nerve cells—you know what *they* do:
Take info to the brain, where can be found
A place that translates a billion sounds.

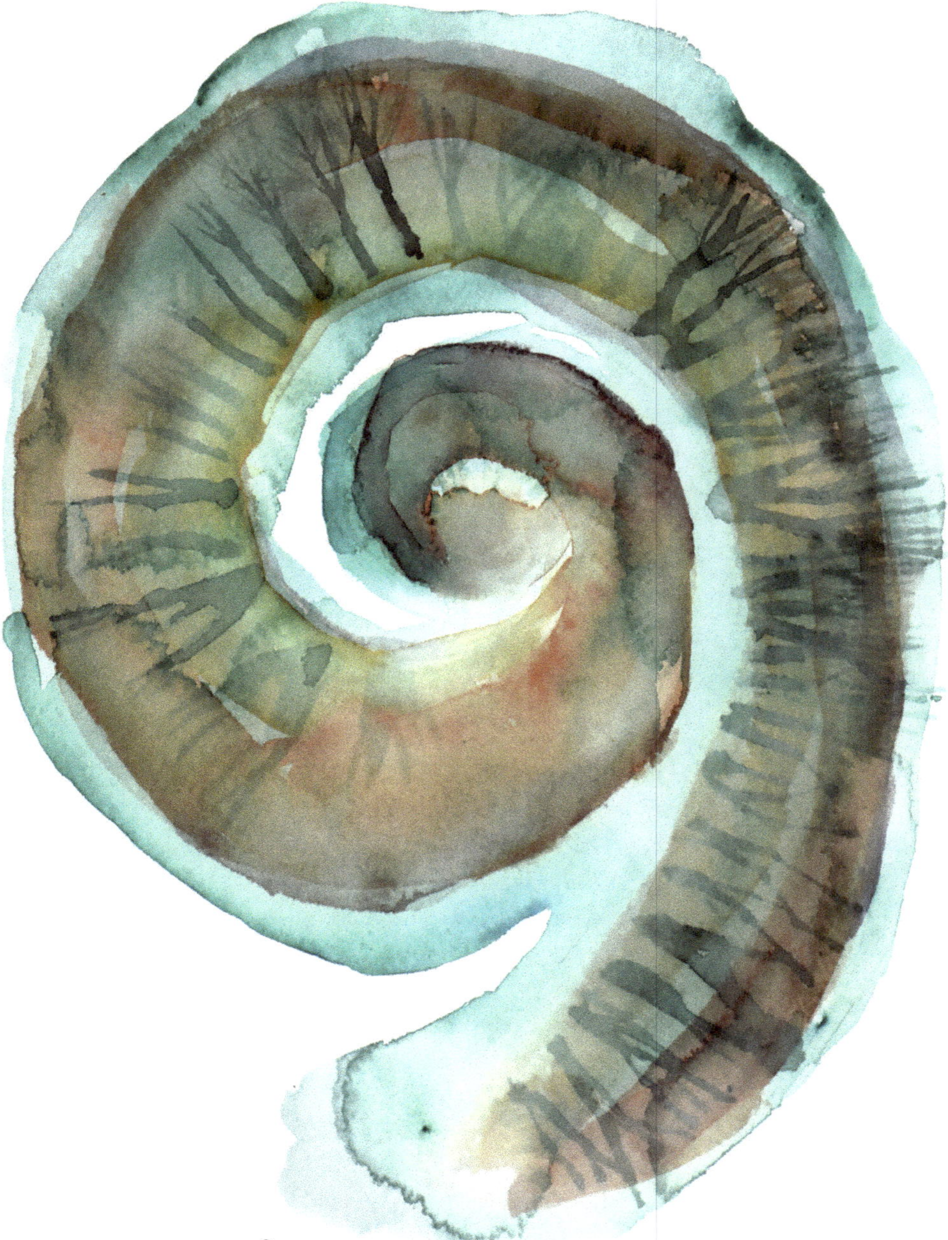

The Cochlea
9x12 Watercolor
2015

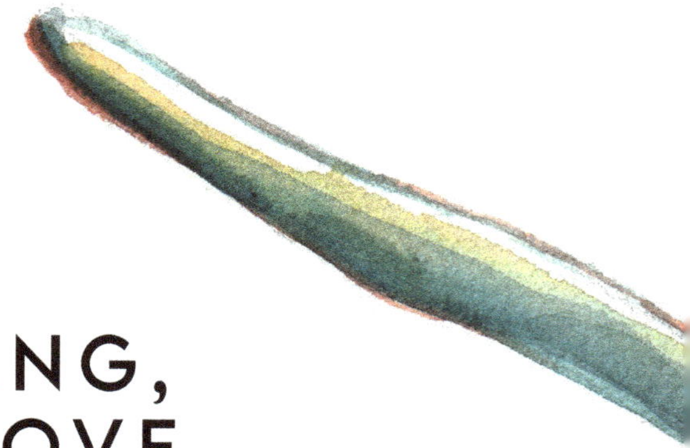

A BANG, A SHOVE AND A SHAKE

Three bones exist for hearing's sake,
Each the size of a dandruff flake.
The malleus and incus
And the stapes all link us
With a bang, a shove and a shake.

First the eardrum thrums like a quake,
And BANG—the malleus awakes!
Shaped like a hammer,
It transmits a rammer
And so starts the bang, shove and shake.

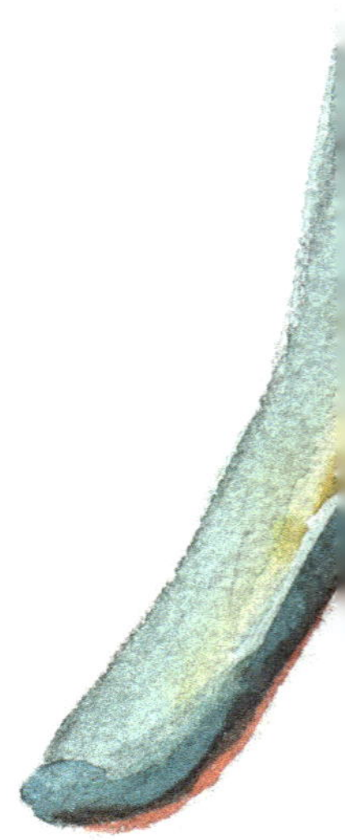

That shove the incus does take,
But it's okay because of its shape.
Formed like an anvil,
All motion it handles,
Continuing the bang, shove and shake.

A big tremble the stapes now makes,
Forcing the inner ear to partake.
Like a stirrup it looks,
A round window, its nook,
And so ends the bang, shove and shake.

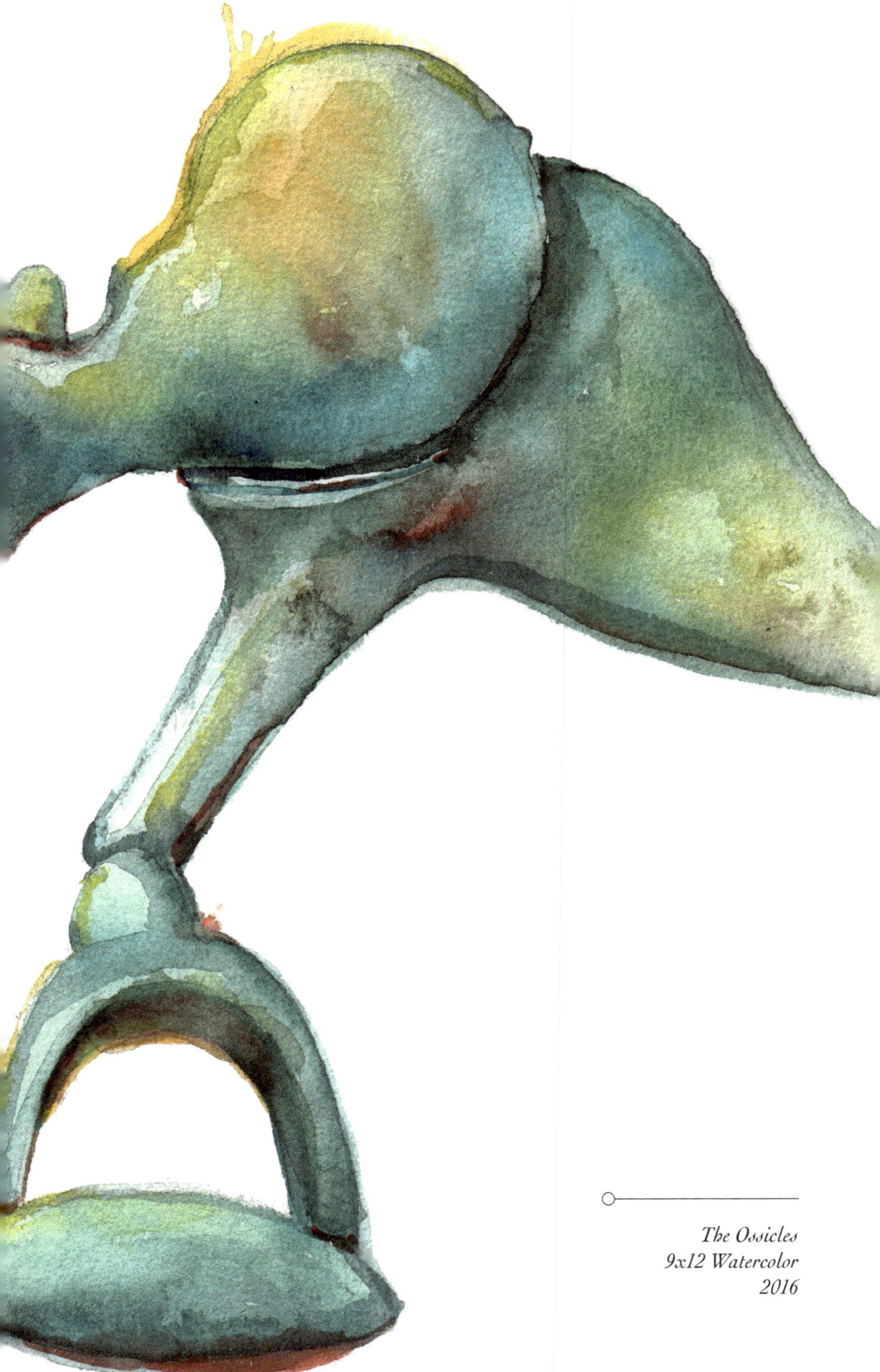

The Ossicles
9x12 Watercolor
2016

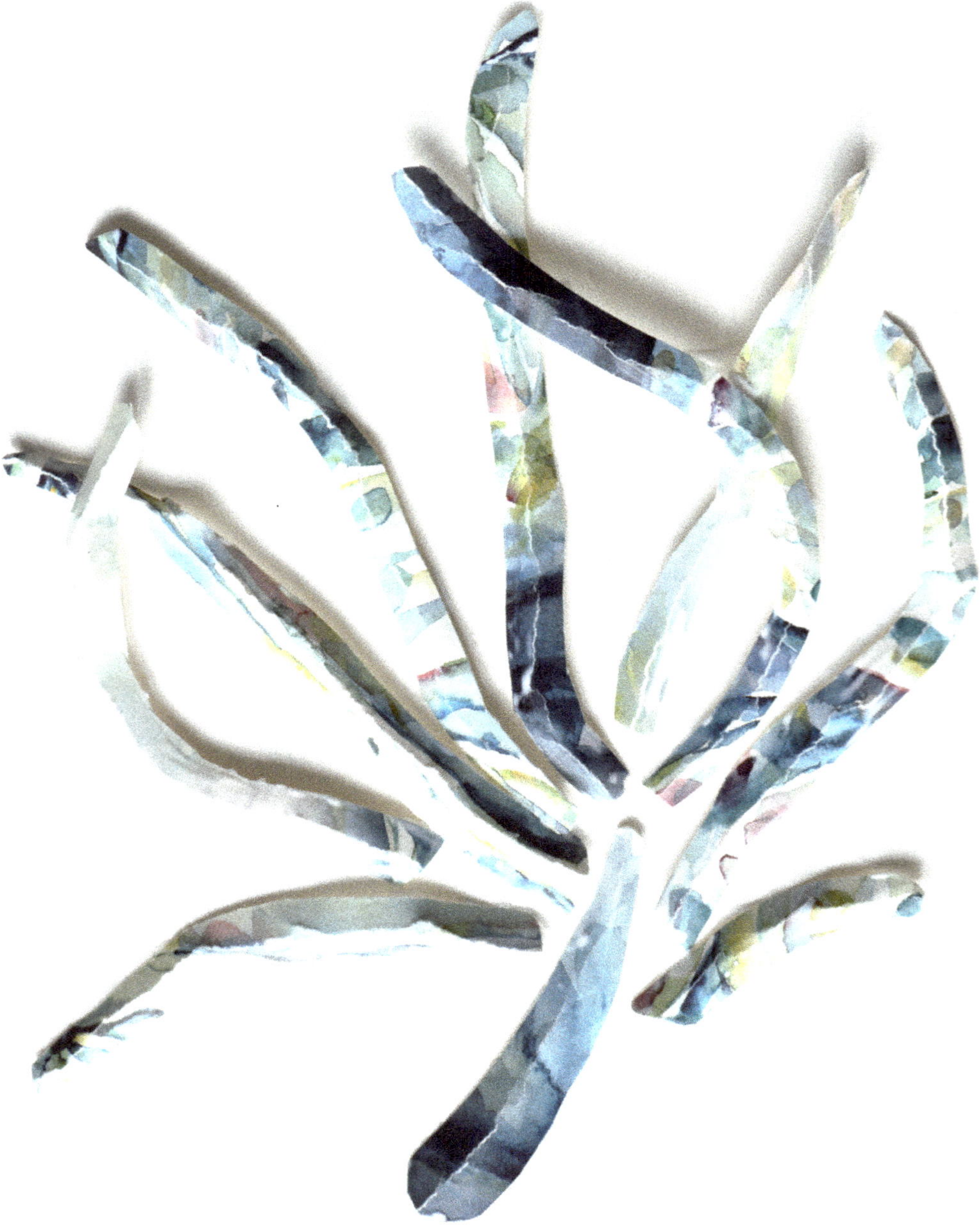

An Olfactory Cell
16x20 Watercolor, Glue, Varnish
2019

I SMELL HOME

I smell home
It smells of nothing
But it is everything
        Everything comforting and warm and safe and peaceful and –
I leave
To explore, to expand, to dream
It smells of everything
But it is nothing
        Nothing comforting and warm and safe and peaceful and –
I return
I smell home
It is everything.

chapter six

PATHOLOGIES & CLINICAL THINGS

"The beginnings and ends of shadow lie between the light and darkness and may be infinitely increased. Shadow is the means by which bodies display their form. The forms of bodies could not be understood in detail but for shadow."

-Leonardo Da Vinci

Antique Stethoscope
9x12 Watercolor
2020

STETHOSCOPE

I get to hear with my little ear
A lub-dub-lub parade.
In a trice, with a simple device,
Through the heart chambers I'll wade.
The handles glisten as I listen
For suspicious sounds to be made.
Like a gentle murmur, which could be a confirmer
That a valve has disobeyed.
Or that awkward rap, that offbeat tap,
When arrhythmia is conveyed.
But while I can hear with my little ear
Things that could make you afraid,
Most of the time it is all sublime,
Just a heartfelt serenade.

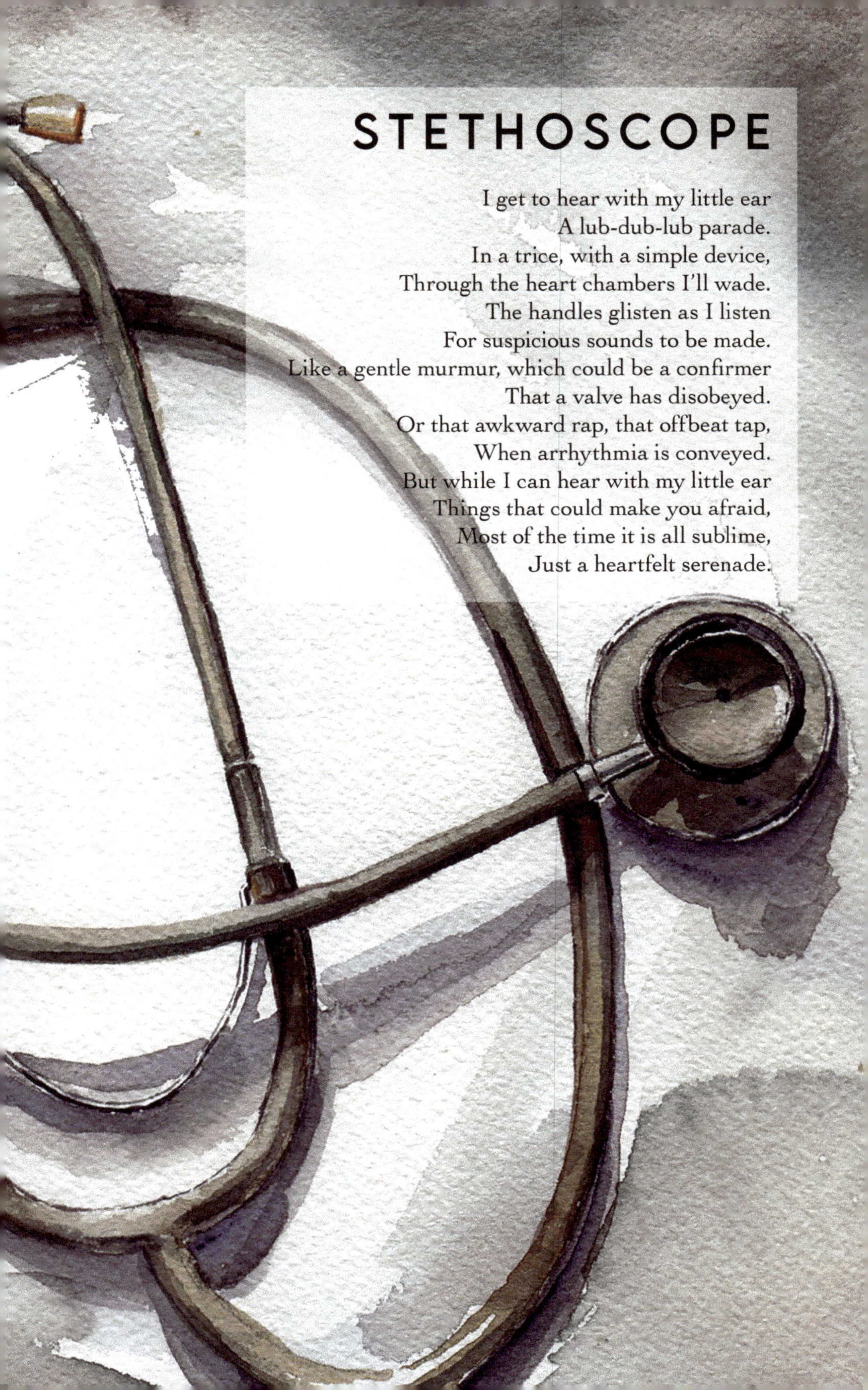

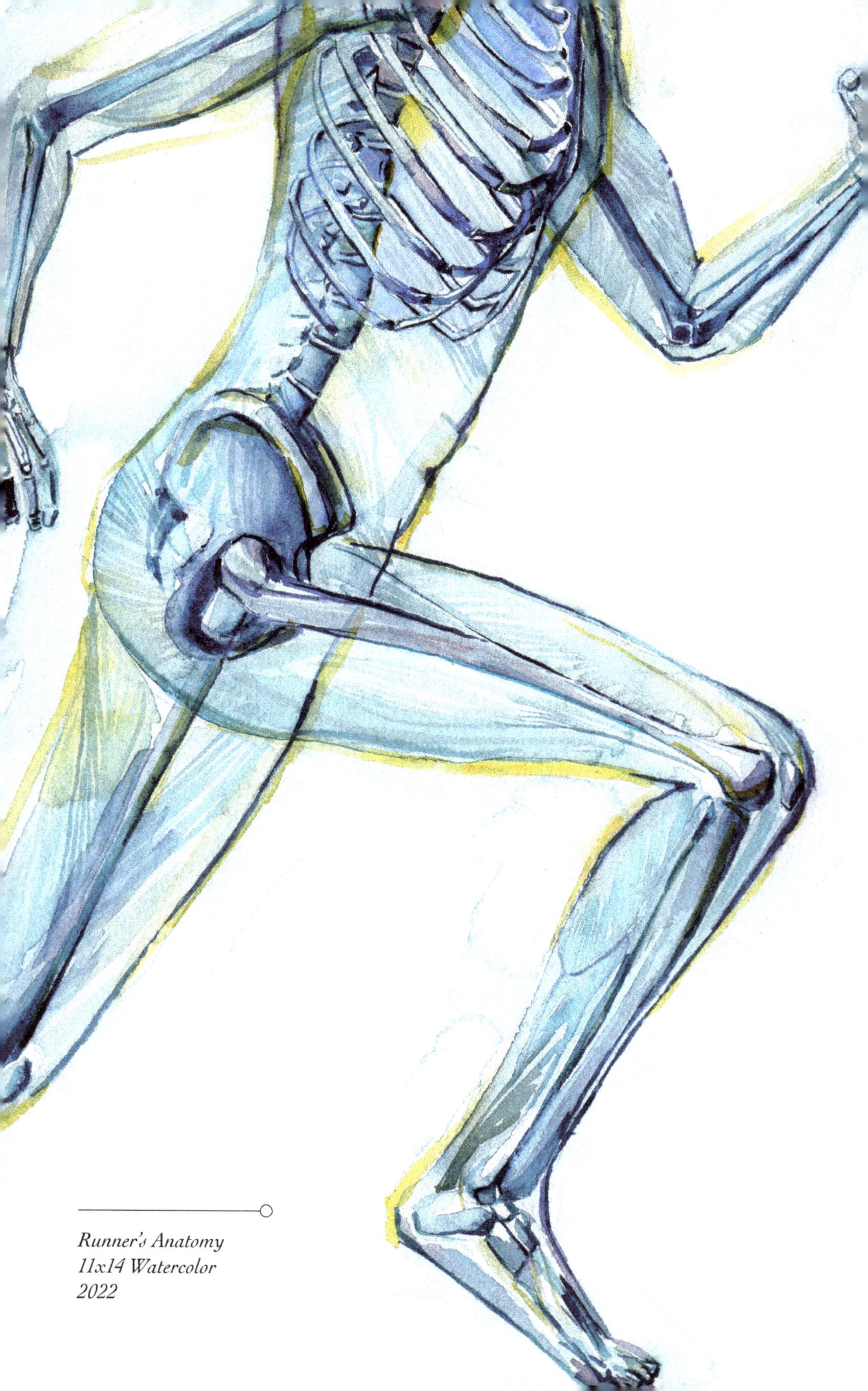

Runner's Anatomy
11x14 Watercolor
2022

EXERCISE

Okay, Body, baby's napping, time to exercise.

Can't we do it when I'm more energized?

NO. Energy begets energy, so c'mon, get up!

I need coffee! Just wait until I have a cup...

Now! Before the opportunity goes awry!

I know I should, Brain, but still, remind me why?

OMG, so many reasons, I don't know where to start..

**sip* I can't wait to hear, Brain; you're so smart.*

Well, I do try. So first, you know it burns calories.

So that I can make my dream body a reality?

Exactly! And it boosts high density lipoproteins.

You know I have no idea what that means.

That's good cholesterol that makes your blood run smoothly.

So less risk of heart disease? That soothes me.

Indeed! And it gets more oxygen to places that need it.

And I get more energy in the process? OK, I see it.

It also stops diseases, for which I have details—

No! No need to list them all, just send me an email!

Best of all, it gives you a high with its chemical boost.

Probably not as good as the one my coffee produced.

Wait a minute... have you just been procrastinating?

No, no, brain, I find lipoproteins just fascinating.

All right, nice try, but that's enough lying.

Uh oh, gotta go, I think I hear the baby crying!

RHEUMATOID ARTHRITIS

Bonjour capitaine, any enemies causing a stir?
—No, everything going along swimmingly, sir.

Sacre bleu! Invaders! I sense zey are near!
—But I swear, sir, we are in the clear!

No, no, release ze troops, or we are doomed!
—Won't that cause a bigger wound?

Tout suite! Or I'll have you court-martialed for delay!
—Okay, okay, sir, then I am on my way.

Captain's Log
Once again, the captain's gone insane.
He thinks he's French and he won't refrain
From raising all troops from their quarters
And rushing them off to the joint borders.
There's no need, I tell him, no enemies are near
But my words never seem to reach his ear.
And I don't want to be charged with dreaded mutiny,
I fear I would perish under such scrutiny.
So I'll comply with his ill-fated request,
Rushing off T-cells at the general's behest.
But I know the damage I cause for his sake,
Fires of inflammation will ignite in our wake.
I weep for the thickening synovial fluid
My tears an echo of it, before it was ruined.
As I ruminate on the joints' lamentable plight,
I know I won't be sleeping tonight.

Rheumatoid Arthritis
11x14 Watercolor
2021

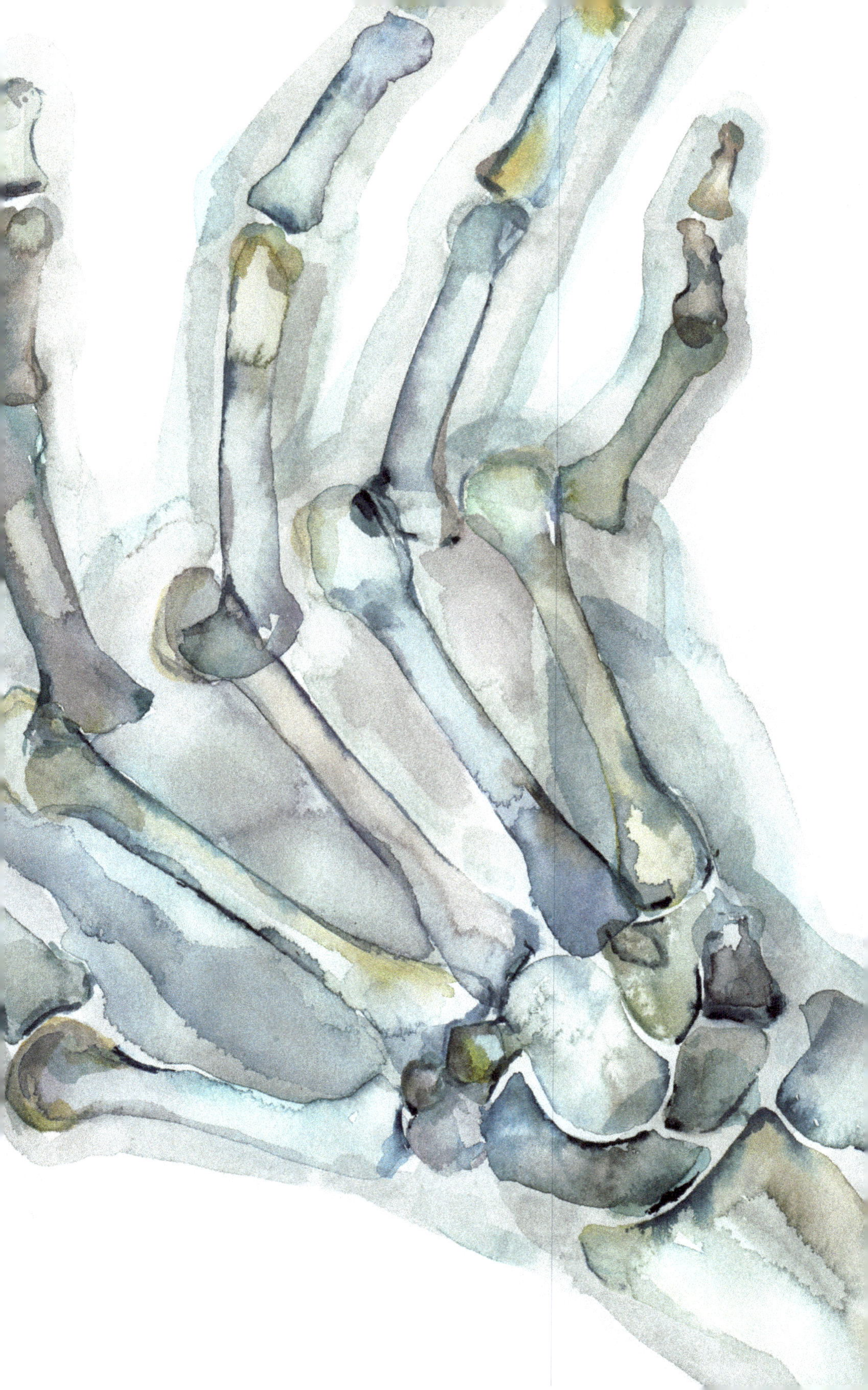

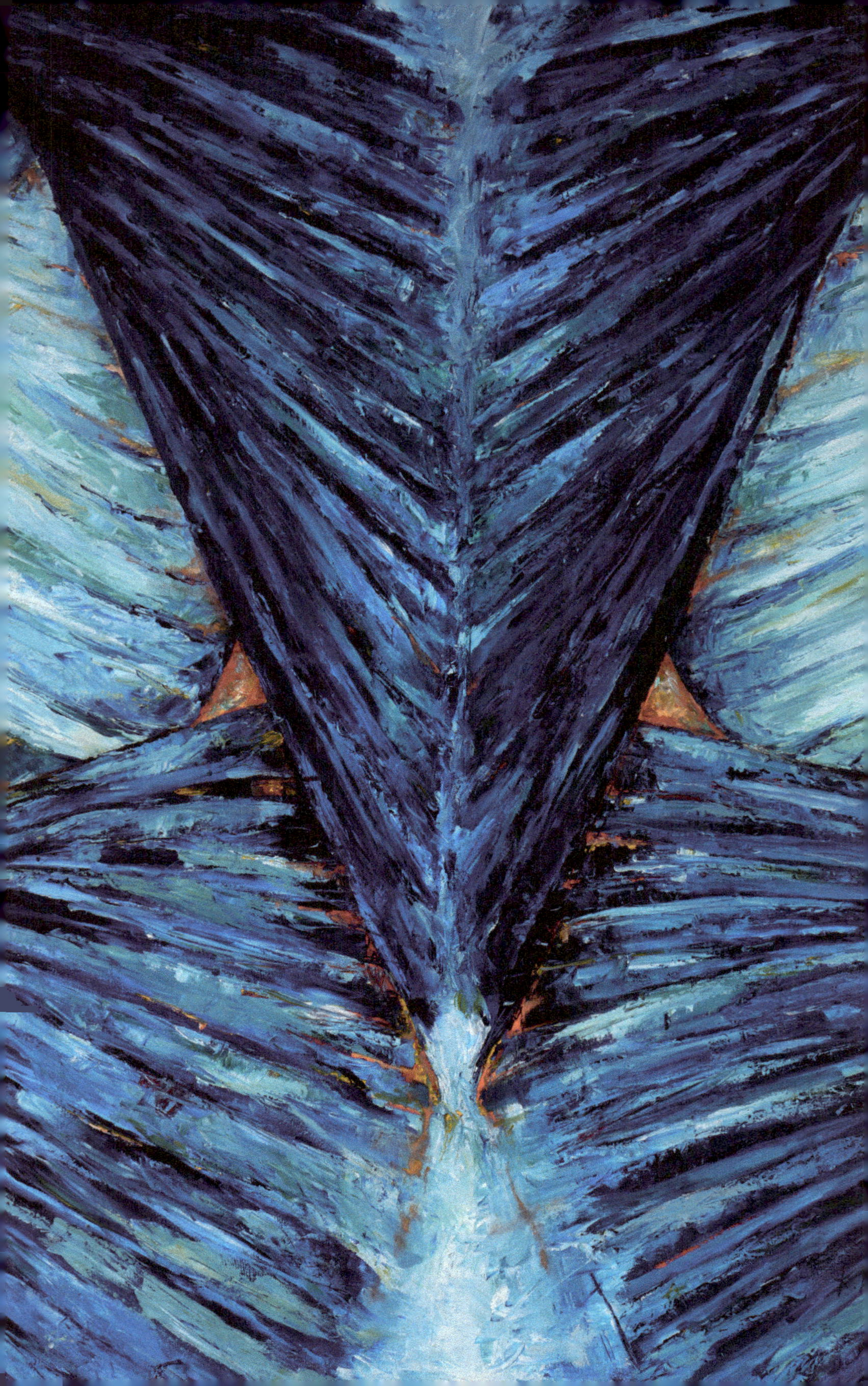

TRIANGLE OF AUSCULTATION

Listen...
Do you hear
The lung's music tracks?

When you
Place your ear
Near that hollow on the back?

A muscle region
That has
A thinner formation,

A valley
Known as
The Triangle of Auscultation.

Triangle of Auscultation
36x48 Oil on Canvas
2017

MONSTER

When cells perpetually proliferate,
Whether in breast or skin or your prostate,
A monster starts to activate,
Using your body to germinate.
Its tentacles reach with added weight,
Stealing resources from every strait,
A kraken that is full of hate,
Tempting the soul to abdicate.

But you have weapons in your arsenal,
Ready to jump into the brawl.
Like potiony, poisonous chemicals
That bring their own nauseous squall.
Or beams of intense energy walls
That slow the monster to a crawl.
But when despair and fear enthrall,
Hope and prayer work best of all.

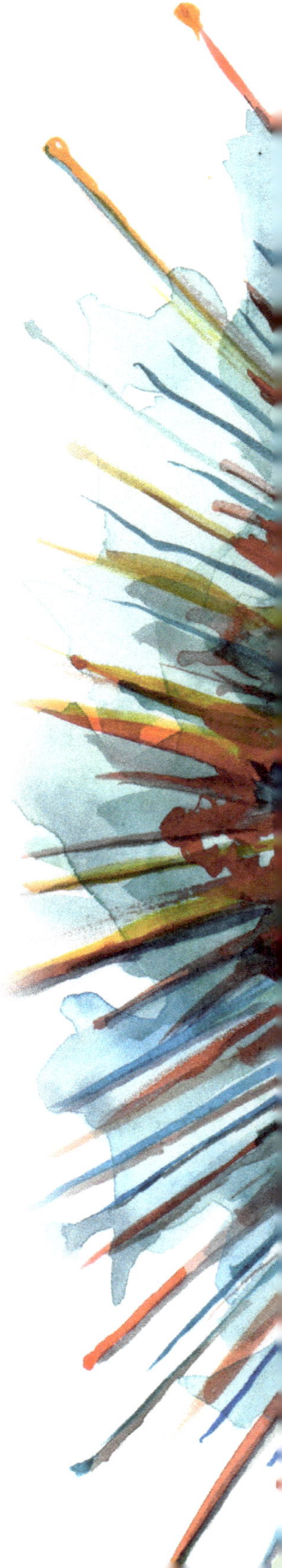

A Cancer Cell
9x12 Watercolor
2018

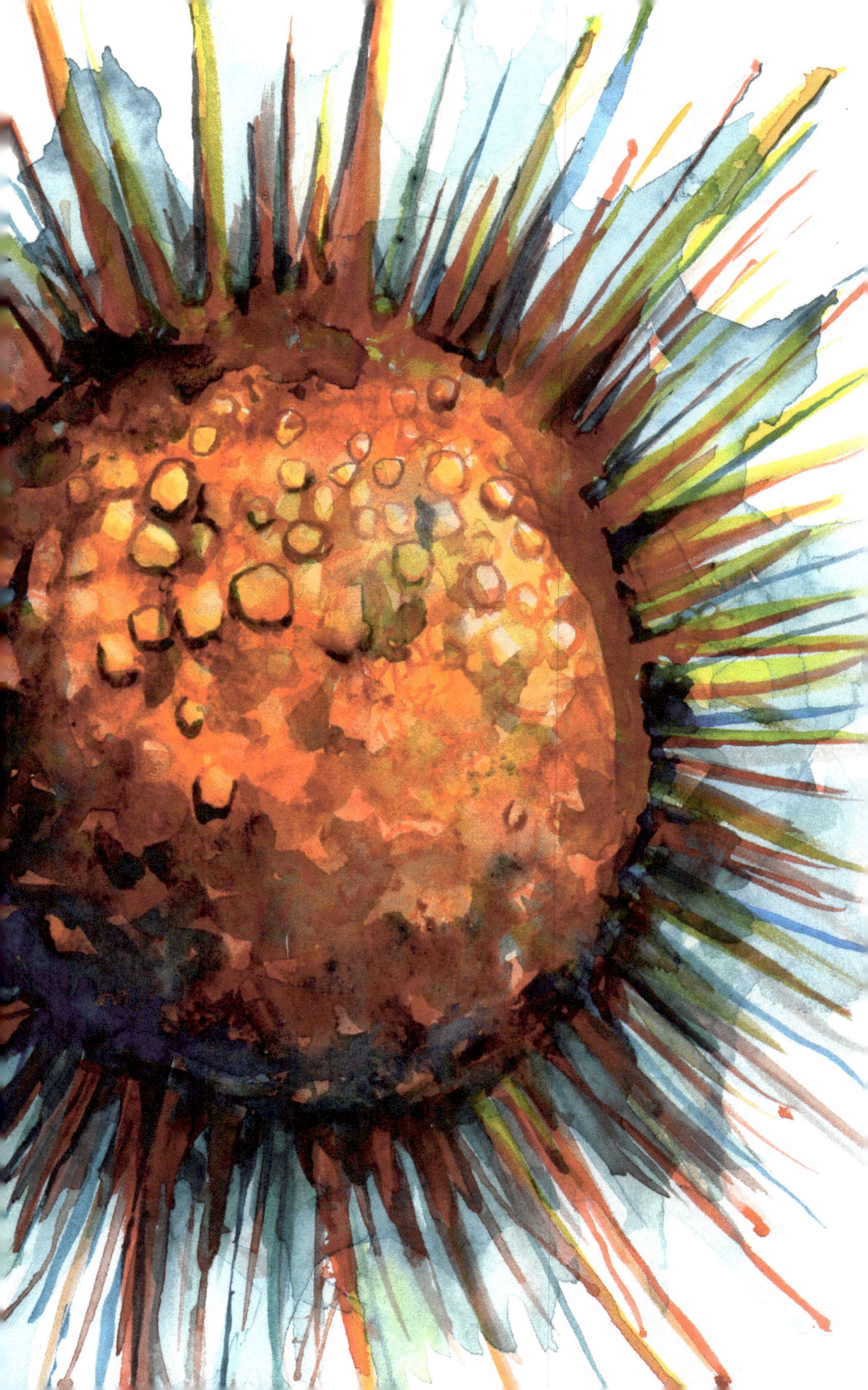

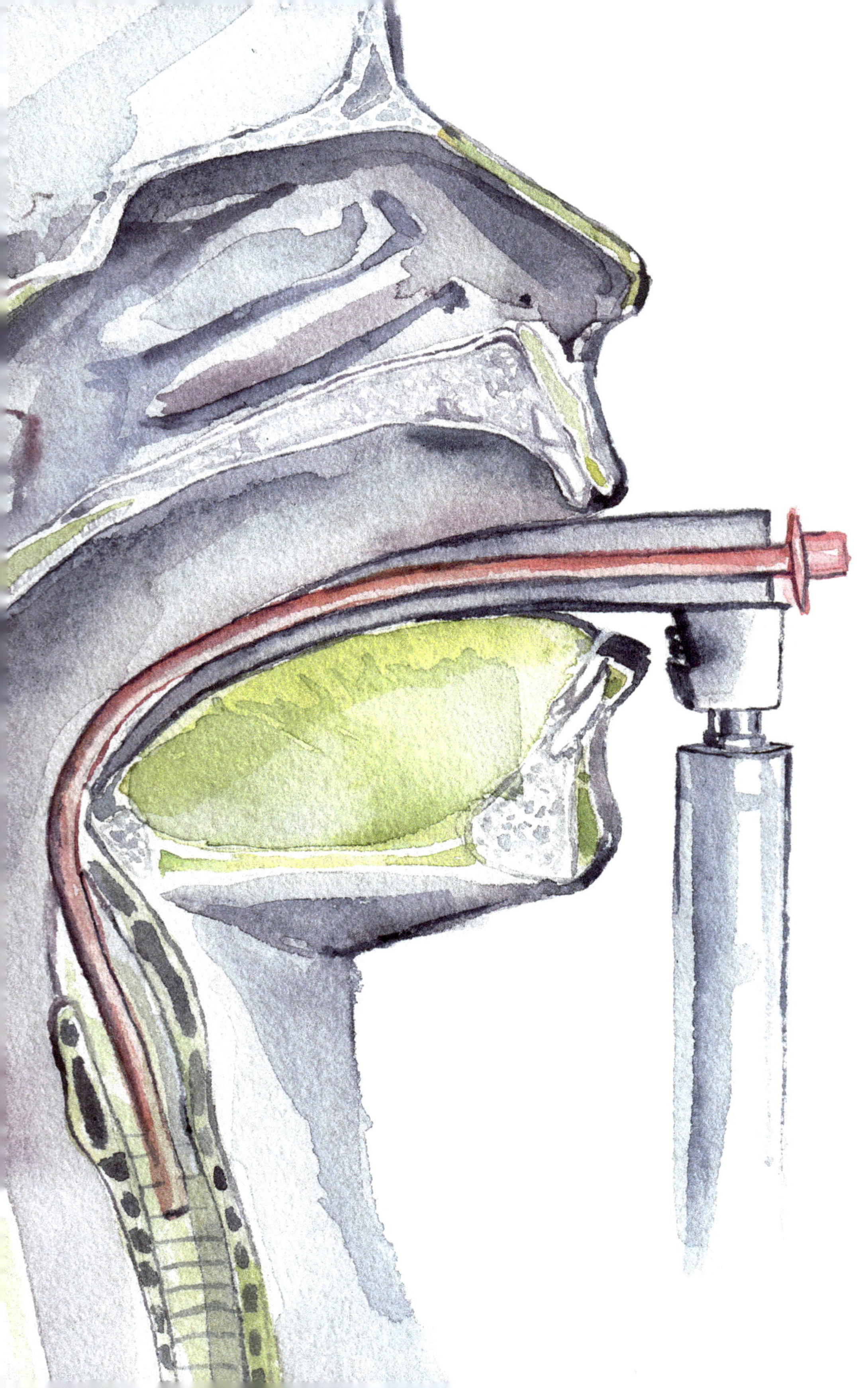

INTUBATION STATION

Welcome to intubation station!
Where the breathing train goes through town.
For when the lungs take a vacation,
The endotracheal tube must go down.

Time to roll out of intubation station!
For the laryngoscope has cleared the road
But watch out for that bifurcation
At the epiglottal abode.

A cheer goes up at Intubation Station!
For you've found the tracheal track.
Now you can give the lungs inflation
And roll the laryngoscope back.

Intubation
8x10 Watercolor
2024

DIABETES I

For Brooke

In diabetes one,
The pancreas is done
With providing an insulin swell.

Without that special stuff,
Dealing with sugar gets rough,
As it can't get into your cells.

Then the sugar stays in your blood
Where it can cause a flood
Of dangerous health issues.

Outside insulin is necessary,
Using a needle as an emissary,
So sugar can reach your tissues.

So when you take a bite
Of something that causes delight
Make sure your insulin is near.

And while diabetes one
Isn't always fun,
You are rocking it, my dear.

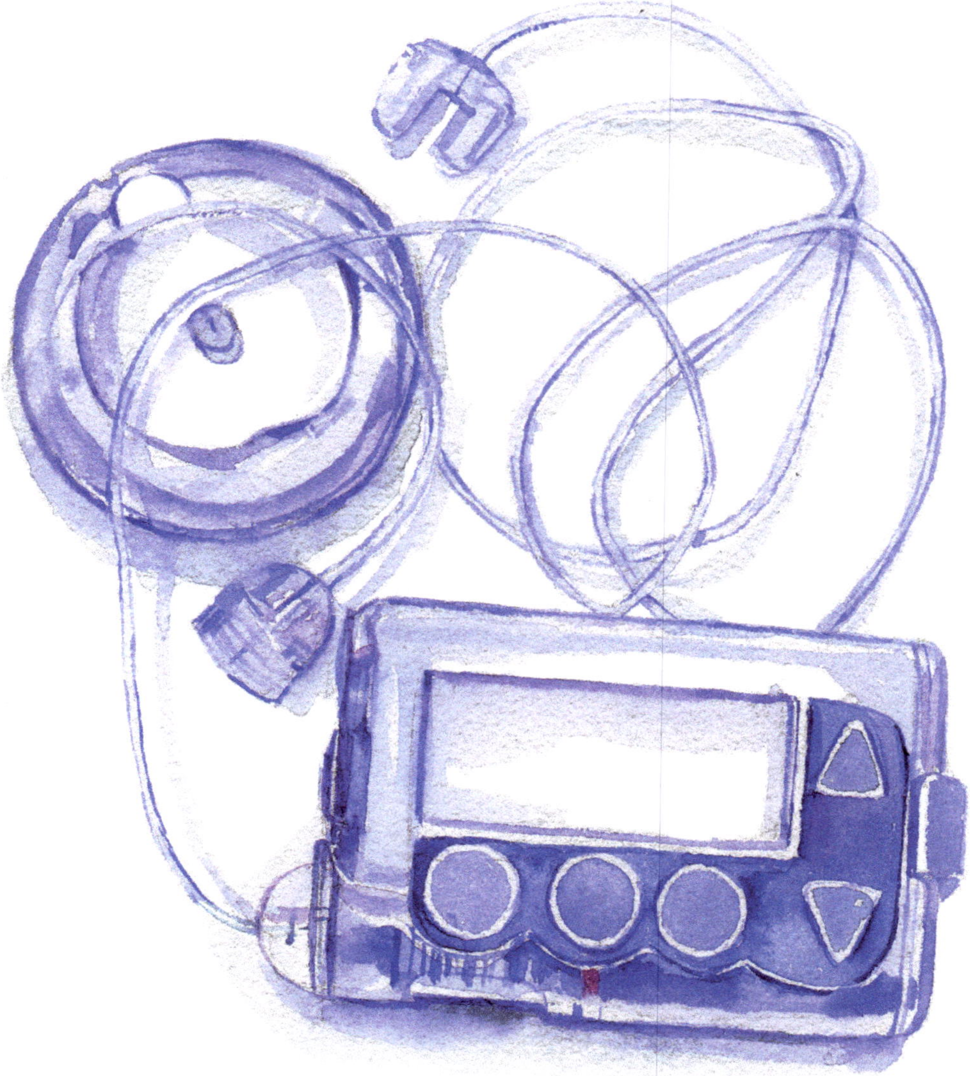

Insulin Pump
8x10 Oil on Canvas
2024

THE LONG GOODBYE

For my dad

His thoughts are leaves,
Swirling around,
Then drifting down,
Landing forgotten
In the rain.

His mind unweaves,
Memories slipping,
Cognition dripping,
Through the perforations
In his brain.

I am bereaved,
As he drifts away,
More each day,
The long goodbye.
My soul drains.

Mind in Pieces
30x40 Mixed Media
2023

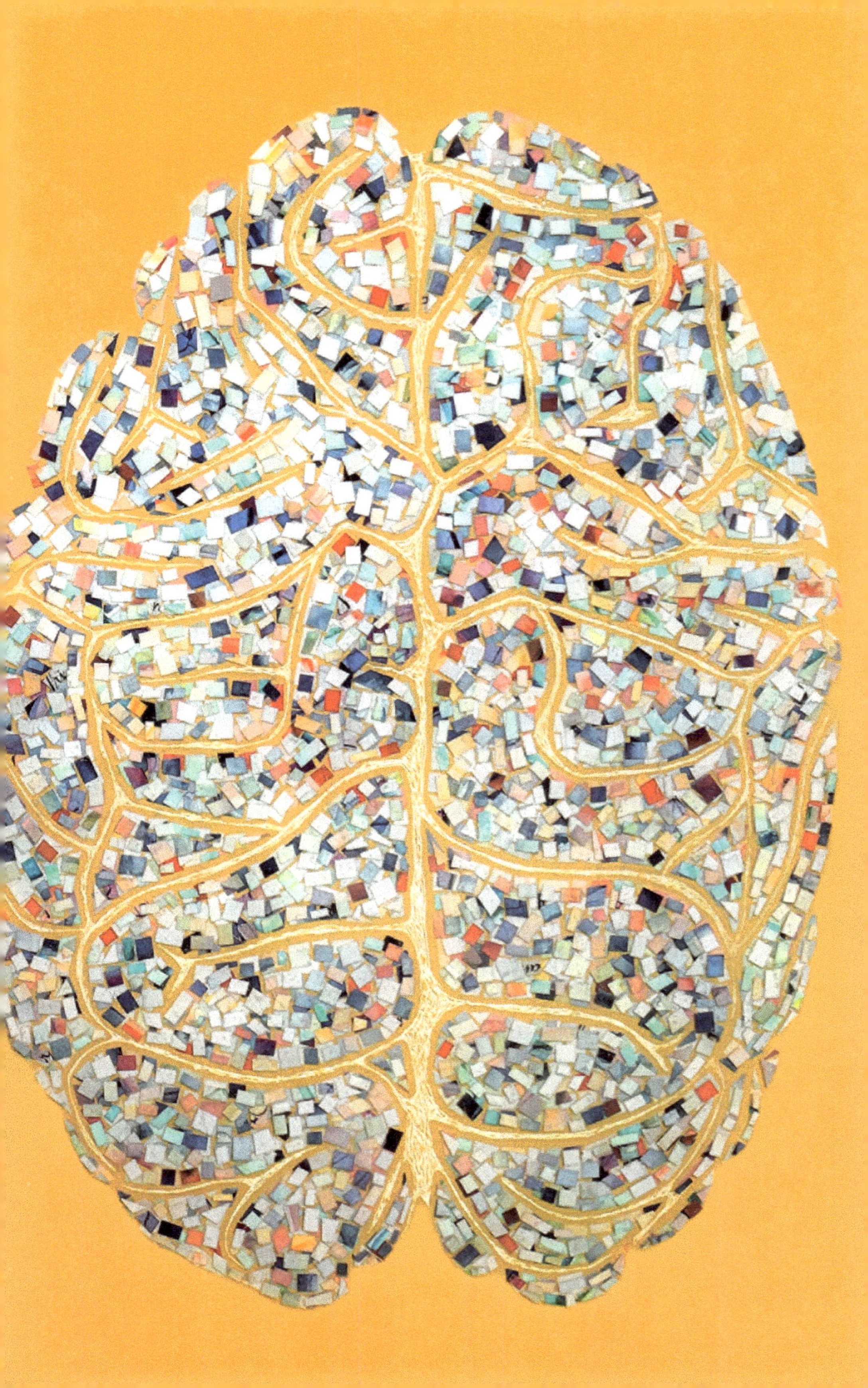

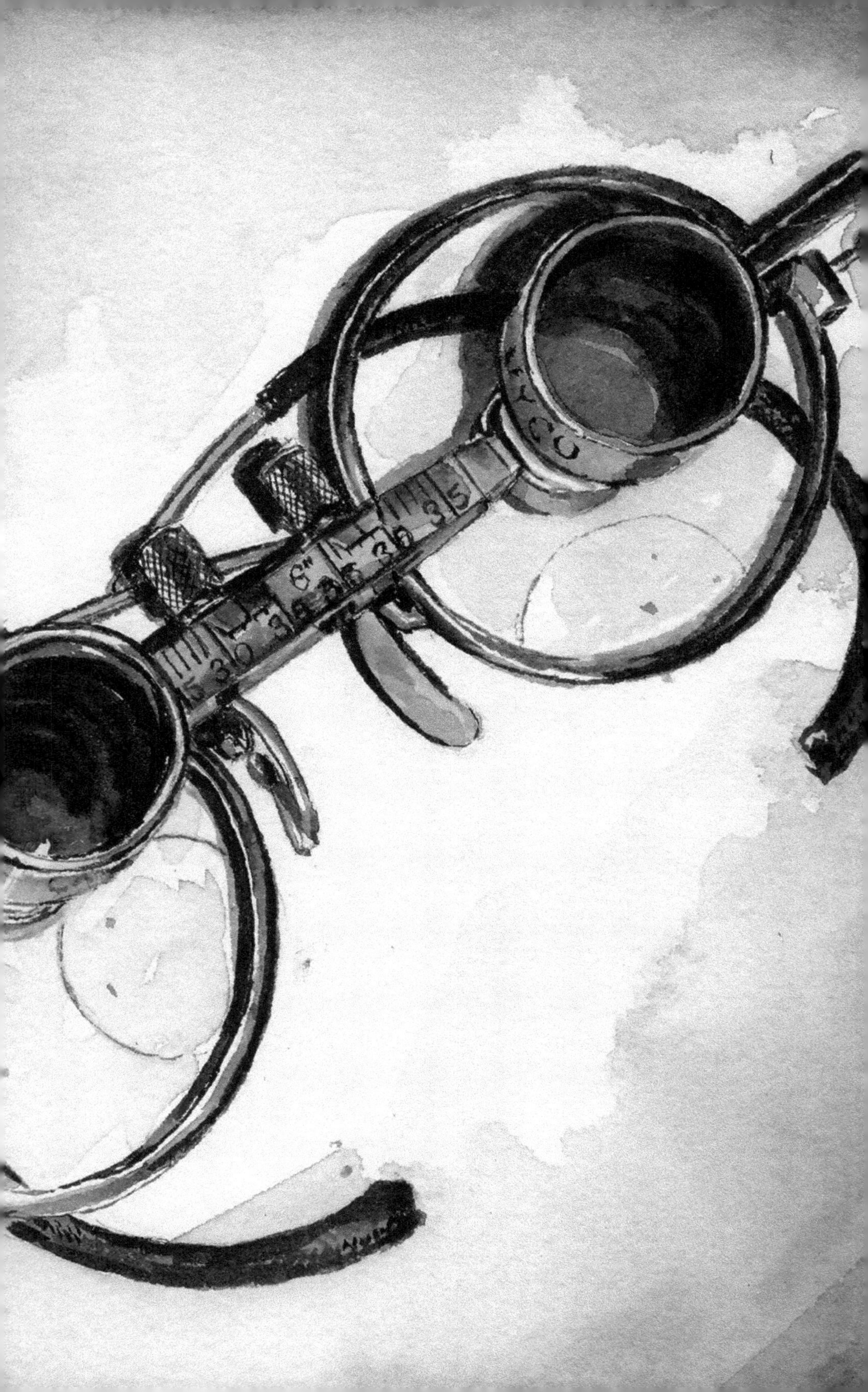

AWESOMESAUCIN' LOUPES

In the dark old days of dentisting
I'd've had to squint and lean and stoop.
But that's no problem anymore
All thanks to my awesomesaucin' loupes.

Like rad, hands-free binoculars
That provide the perfect snoop
Of the dank, dark cave of the mouth...
How great are these awesomesaucin' loupes?

Lenses on lenses with a bionic flare,
Steel earpieces that never droop
A clip-on light to bring it together,
You need some awesomesaucin' loupes.

Once the metal skims my nose
I feel like an army ranger troop
I now surgerize with military precision...
I love my awesomesaucin' loupes.

Antique Loupes
10x10 Watercolor
2022

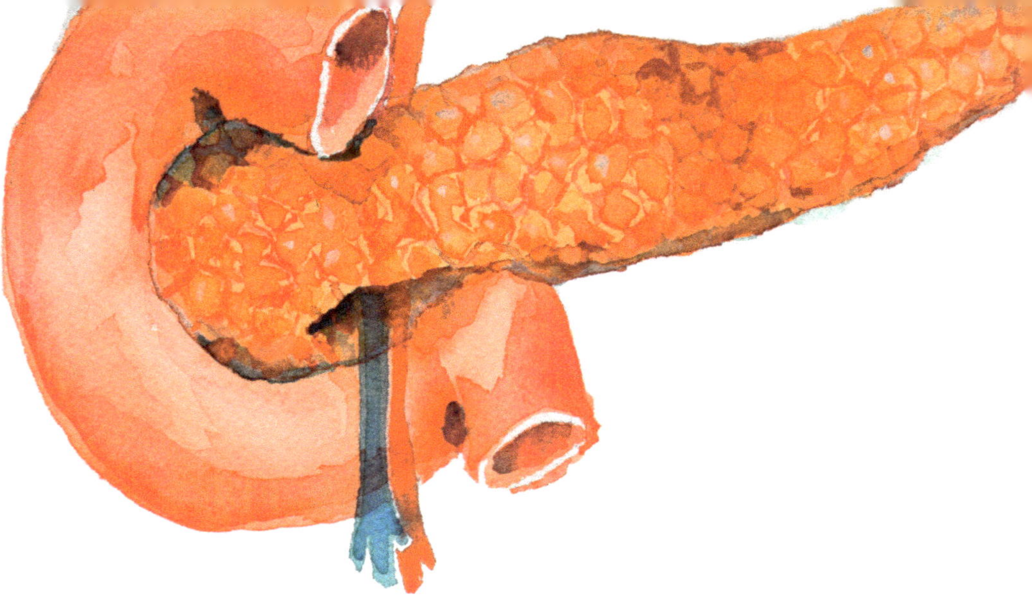

DIABETES II

In diabetes two,
It's the cells that are through
Responding to insulin's effects.

While insulin is still made,
The cells just throw shade,
So in the blood the sugar collects.

Since the insulin's been subverted,
The pancreas should be alerted,
Then it knows it should make more.

In type two this won't occur,
So there's not much to deter
Blood sugar spikes galore.

The thing about this version,
When cells have insulin aversion,
Shots won't provide any support.

Instead its exercise you need,
And a healthy diet to exceed,
And meds as a last resort.

Pancreas
10x8 Watercolor
2016

chapter six

PATHOLOGIES & CLINICAL THINGS

"Once you have tasted flight, you will forever walk the earth with your eyes turned skyward, for there you have been, and there you will always long to return."

-Leonardo Da Vinci

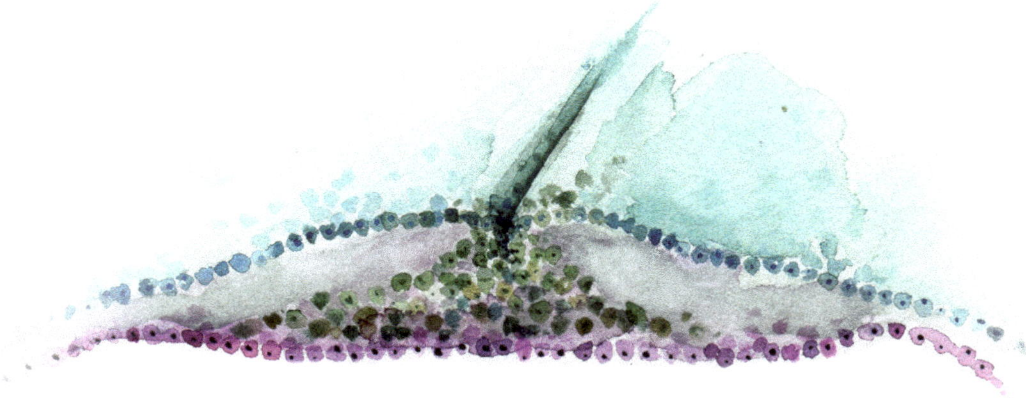

PRIMITIVE STREAK

A disc of cells grows with rapid speed.
Multiplying endlessly, without heed.
At first their squirming seems to be random
But then you see they're moving in tandem.
Pushing and reaching toward the midline,
Where they invaginate into a design.
That indented path the cells seem to seek,
Falling gladly into this primitive streak.
Once there, they move with elegant intention,
Though you'll have to start thinking in three dimensions,
For as they drop down, they spread out here
And along this new axis they form some tiers.
Which is the point of this cellular dance:
The three germ layers, and their advance.
They form a pocket where, deep in the dark,
The genesis of life at last can embark.

Primitive Streak
7x5 Watercolor
2020

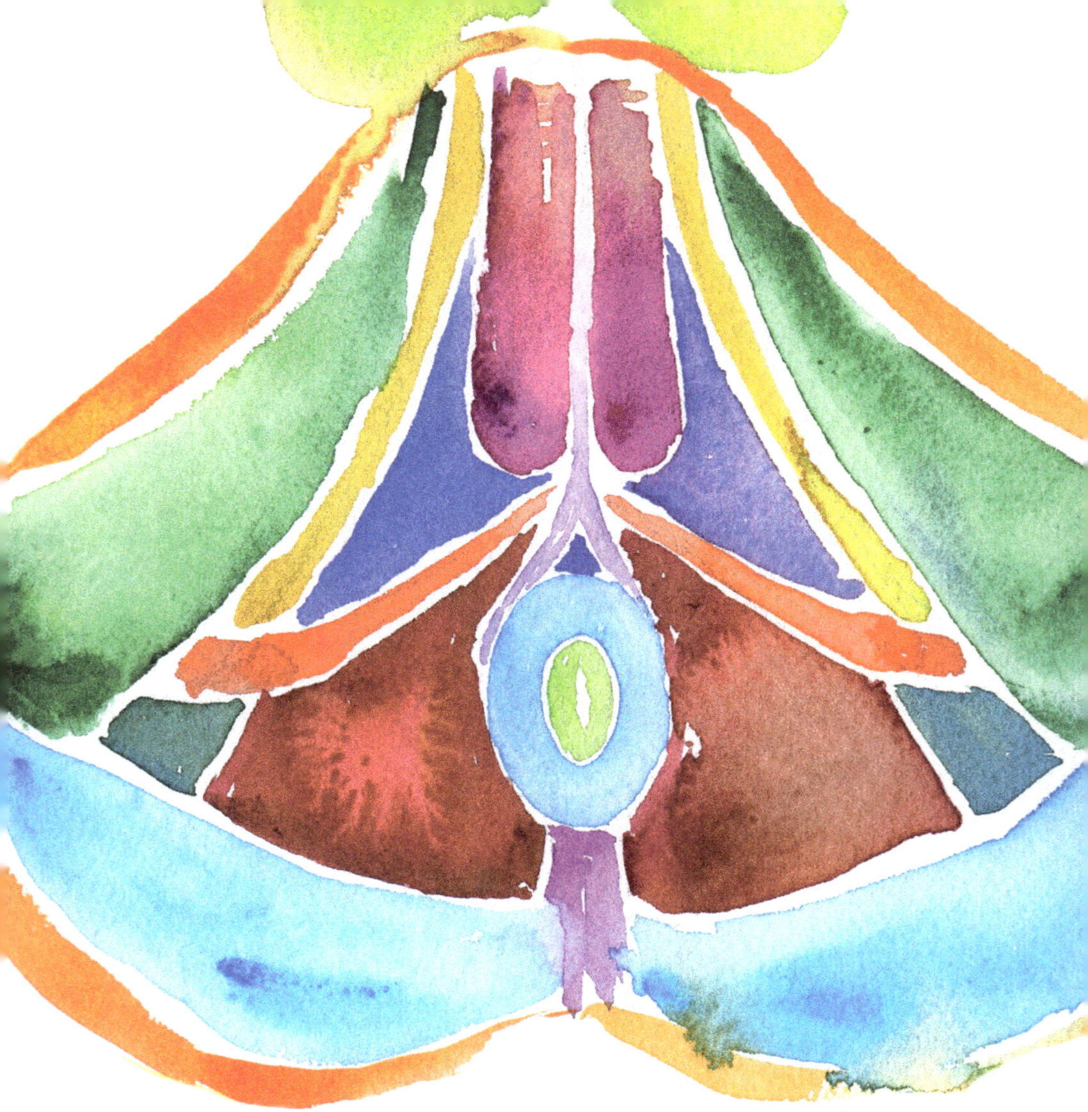

MALE PERINEUM

The perineum is fickle
Hiding behind a man's pickle.
But you'll earn its affection
(And an erection)
If you give it a tickle.

Male Perineum
10x10 Watercolor
2024

CERVIX

The cervix is a plushy portal
Through which a flow of liquid is normal.
Sounds easy, but it lives in fear
Of a day that draws ever-near
When it will have to pass through a mortal.

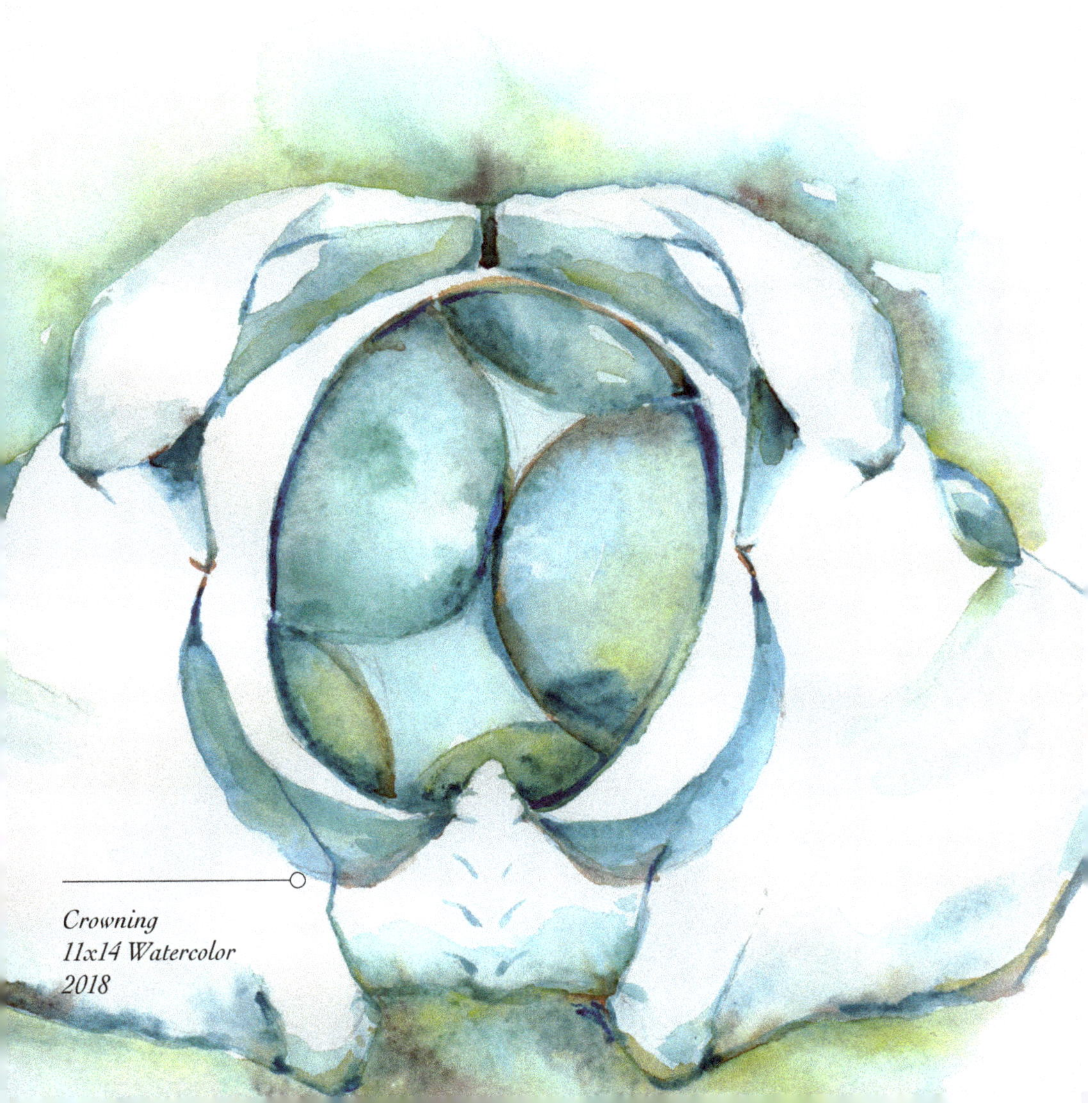

Crowning
11x14 Watercolor
2018

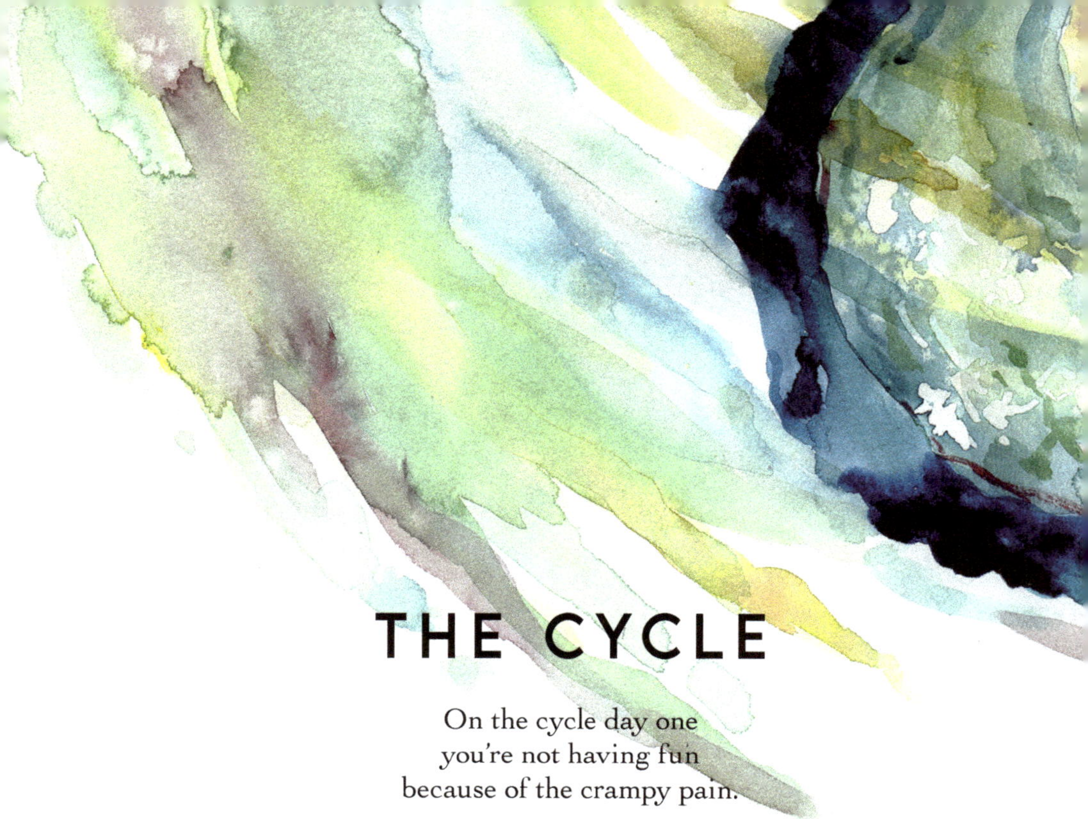

THE CYCLE

On the cycle day one
you're not having fun
because of the crampy pain.

At this point your follicle
is small like a molecule
(follicle is an egg's *fancy* name).

Day 3 through 10 it's developing,
the cells around enveloping
that precious little egg.

Then around day thirteen,
mature it would seem,
because the estrogen no longer lags.

Day fourteen there's a "pop!"
as the egg leaves the shop:
Ovulation is its fate!

This important purge
is caused by a surge
of estrogen and LH.

Ovary and Fimbriae II
30x22 Watercolor
2020

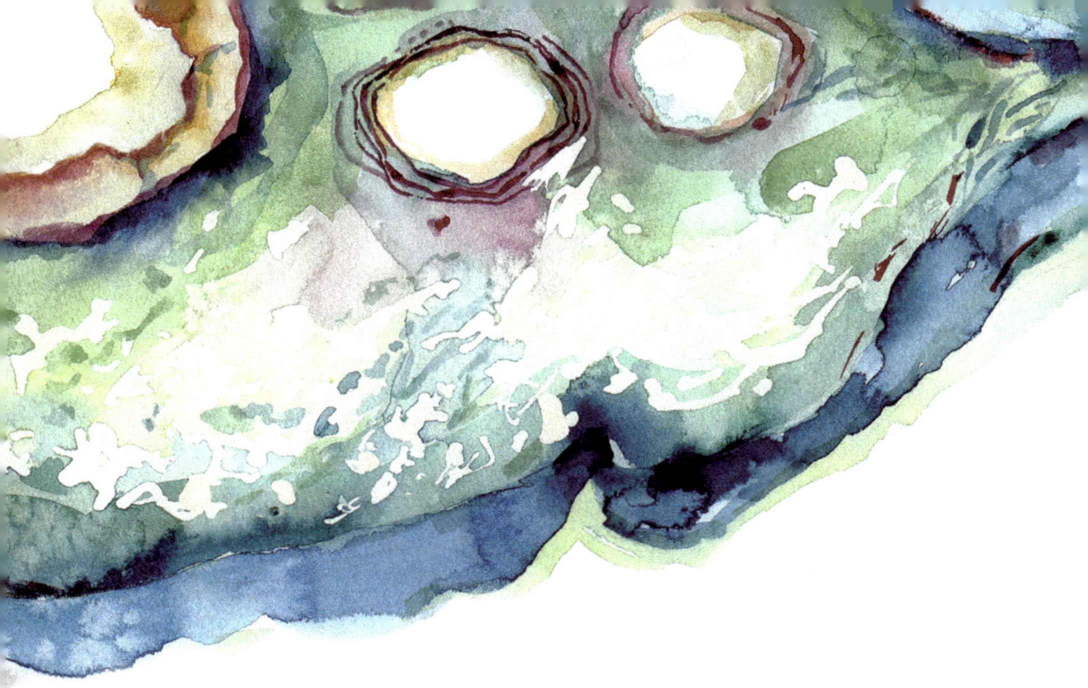

But those hormones do drop
after that pop
and the follicle becomes a new structure.

The corpus luteum it's named,
for progesterone it is famed,
releasing it at this juncture.

Ms. Luteum reigns
for sixteen days
during which PMS makes you crabby.

But by day twenty eight
Luteum gets its fate
and it is a little shabby.

The ovary it will mar
as it turns into a scar,
transforming into corpus albicans.

The hormones now ebb,
though they still weave a web,
and the cycle will begin again.

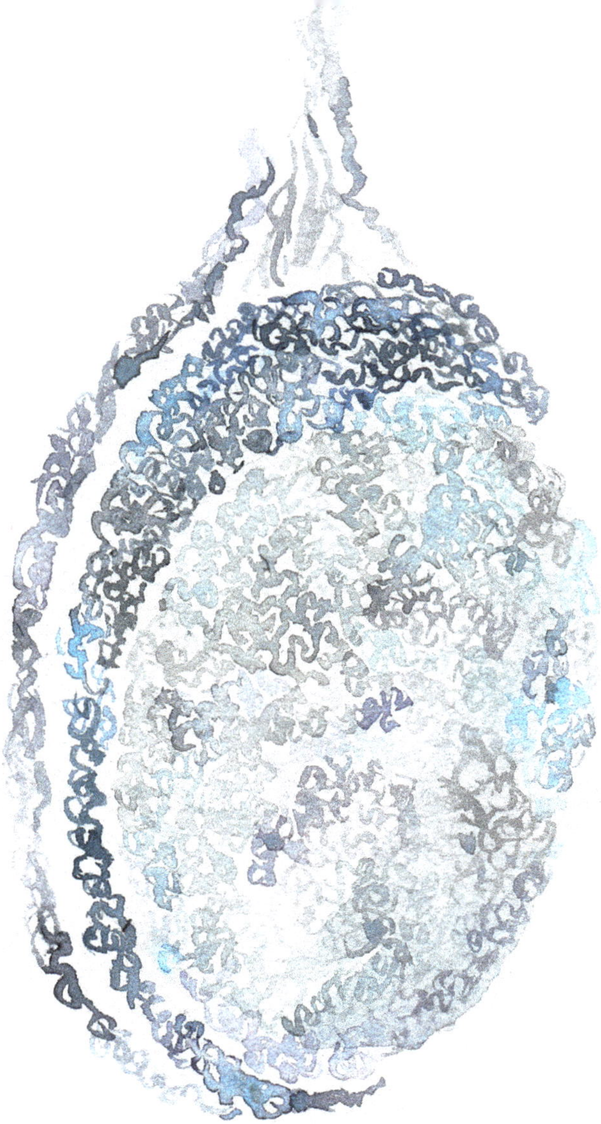

EPIDIDYMIS

A spermatazoa starts out wild
But the epididymis turns it mild.
It goes in a cad,
Comes out half a dad,
Ready to make you a child!

Epididymis
6x9 Watercolor
2024

OVULATION

My estrogen and interest are peaked!
I'm turned on by your manly physique!
Then progesterone drops.
You're no longer as hot.
Sorry—maybe try again in three weeks.

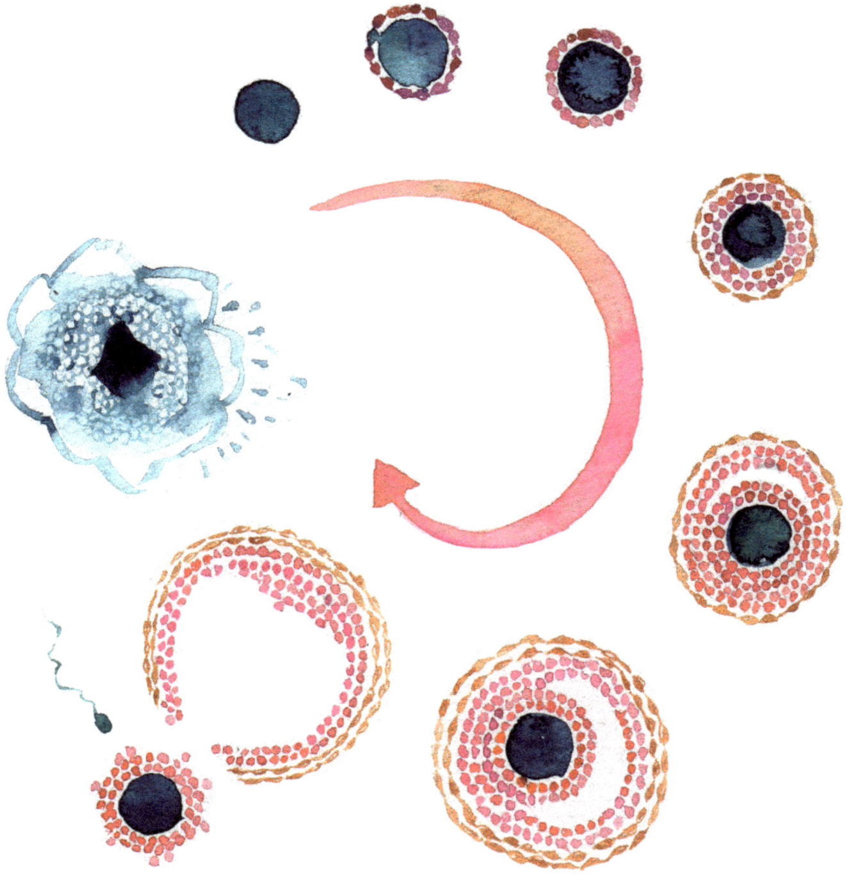

Menstrual Cycle
8x10 Watercolor
2023

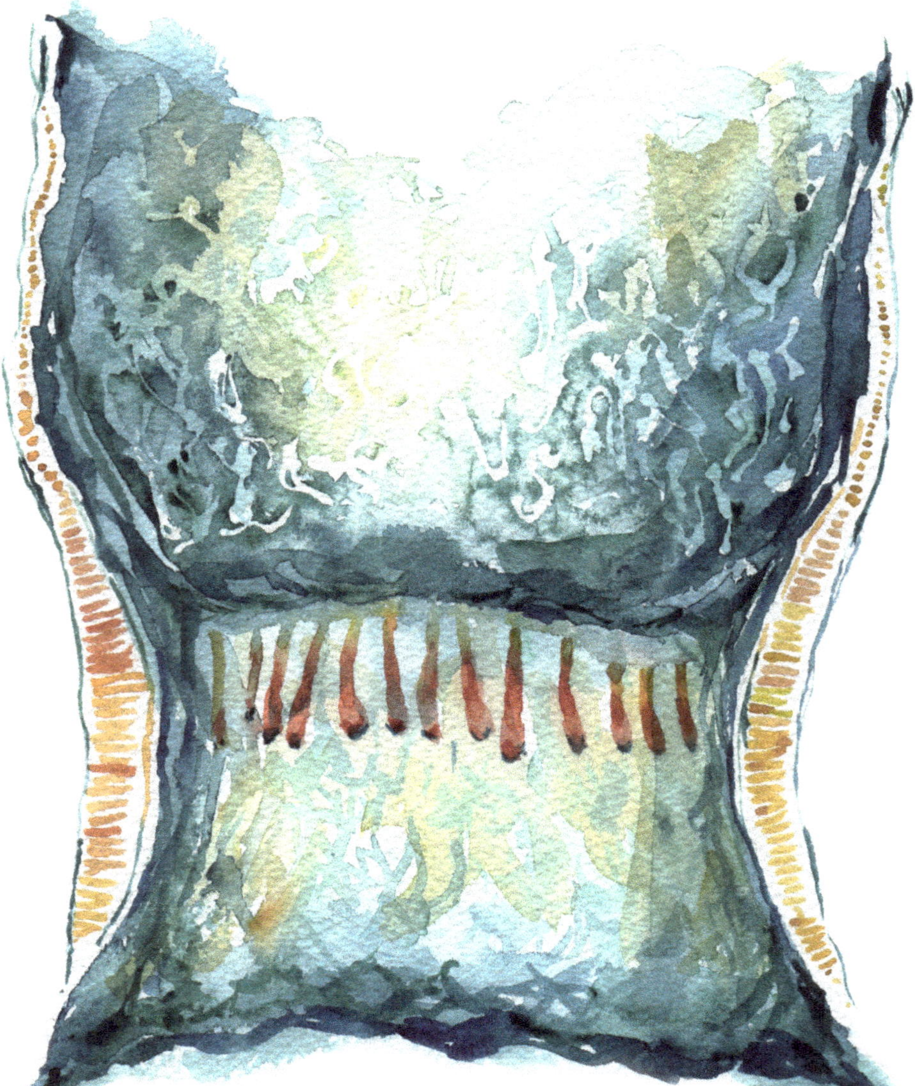

ANAL SPHINCTER

At the end of the colon two muscles cinch tight
The inner one gets to command its own plight.
The outer one you mostly control.
But sometimes it just has to let go...
And ready or not your poop will take flight.

Anal Canal
8x10 Watercolor
2021

TURNING 35

My egg release feels dramatic,
And each month is more traumatic.
For there's not many left,
Which makes me bereft
Now that my eggs are geriatric.

Flower Uterus
9x12 Watercolor
2023

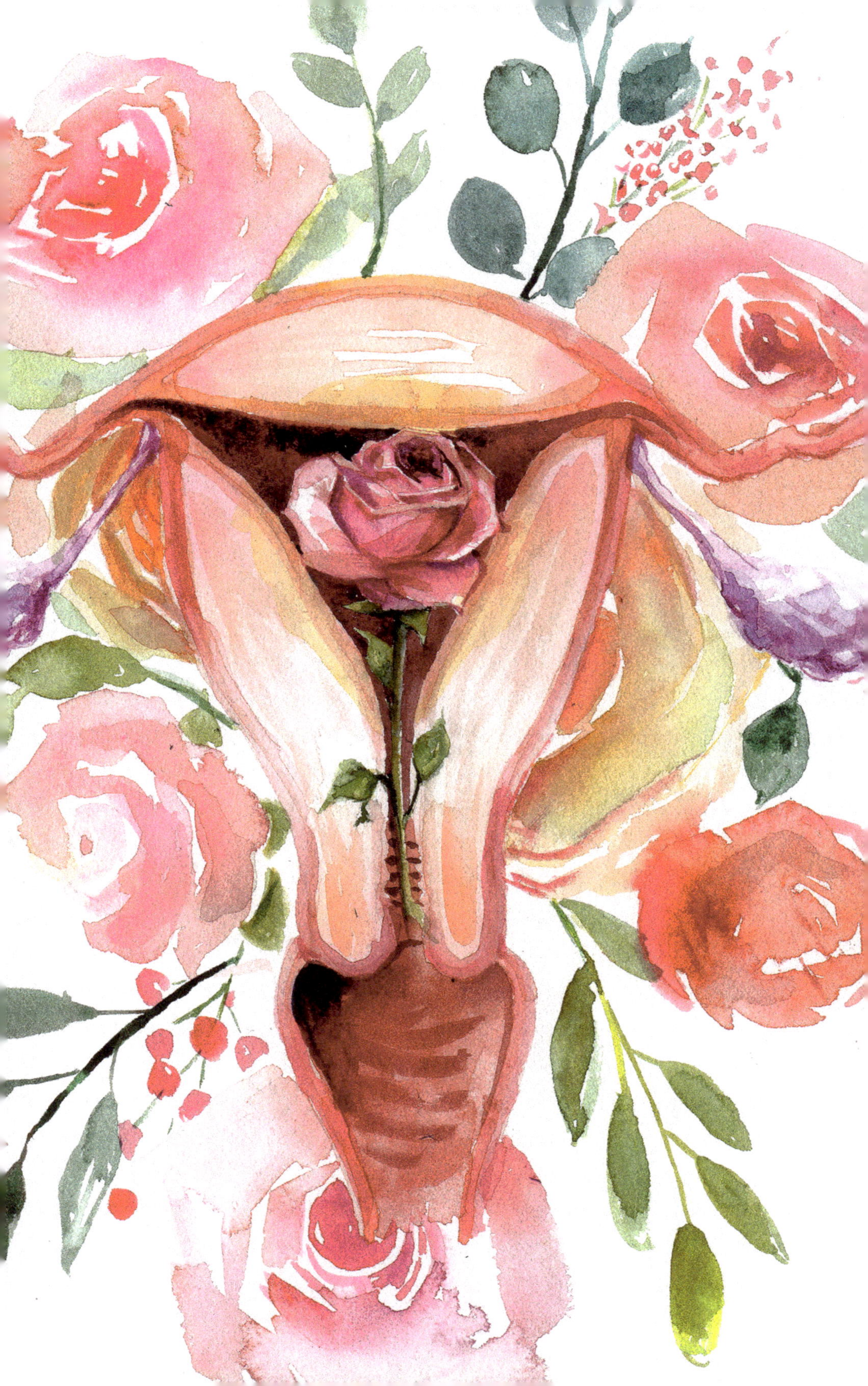

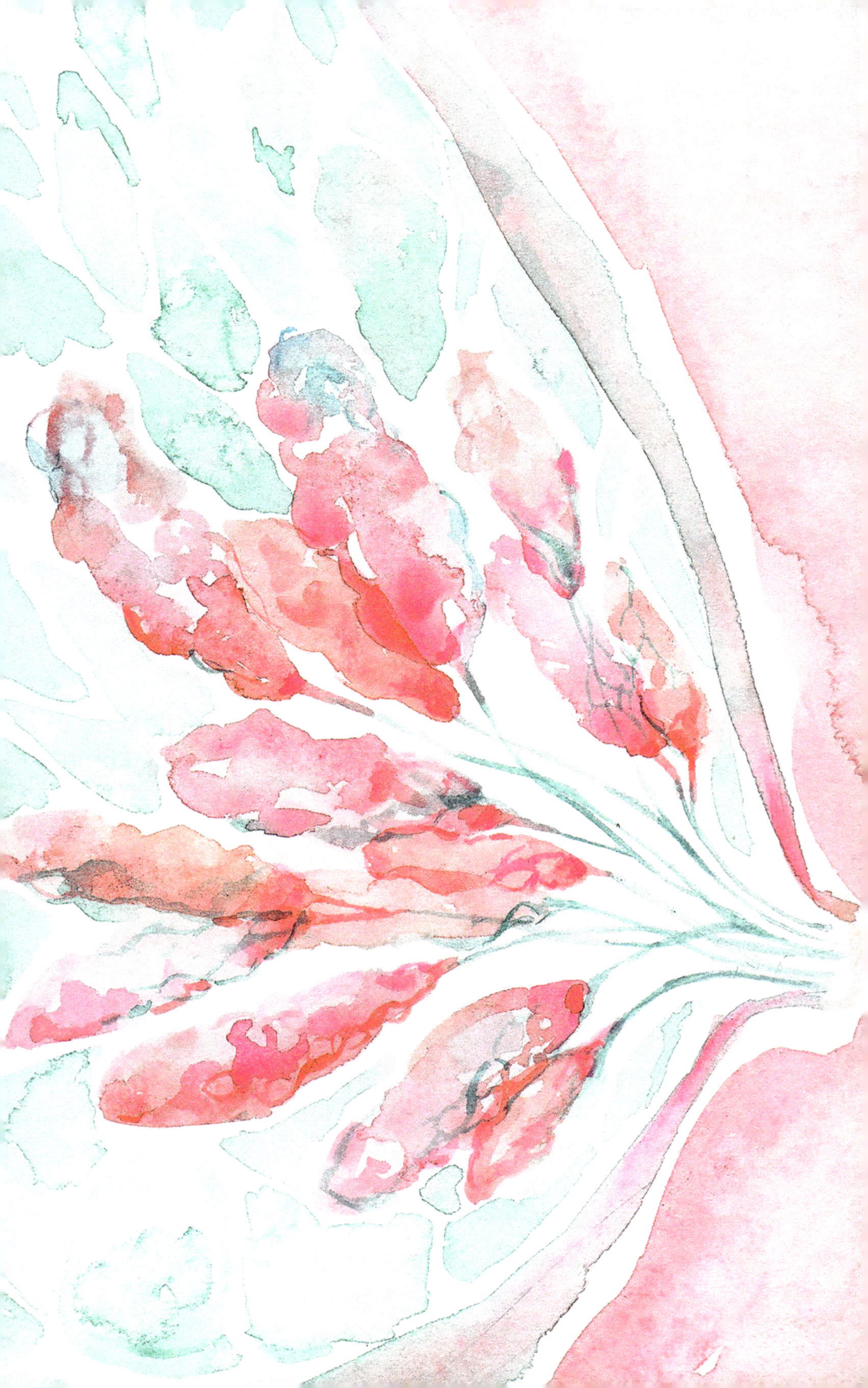

LACTATION

"Momma, how does the baby get fed?"
"I'll tell you the tale as I put you to bed"

Many moons ago, after I'd been amorous
Prolactin gurgled below my hypothalamus.
When the time was right, it released in a rush
Making my breasts engorged, ripe and plush.
But the thing about prolactin is that when it swells,
It releases a potent, magical, mystical spell
That leads to the creation of mother's milk,
Sweet as cantaloupe, smooth as silk.
So when your baby brother clawed his way out
His beverage was ready before he could pout.
But that's not the whole story, it's really just half.
For how do these udders open up to my calf?
It comes from a suckle, his pull on my teat
(Which doesn't hurt much, until he gets teeth).
That motion is like the wave of a wand
And it triggers two hormones to emerge from the pond.
One is prolactin again to replenish,
In order to satisfy your brother's milk fetish.
The other is the chemical called oxytocin
A happy and beloved feel-good potion.
Along with a host of warm fuzzy feelings,
(That, by the way, aids mental healing)
Causes the let-down within these two mountains
And ready or not, my nipples are fountains.
So with two hormones, and a suck that won't rest
Your brother is fed with my magical chest.

"So, dear, is that what you were looking for?"
"I don't want to ask you questions anymore."

Lactation
6x9 Watercolor
2019

chapter seven

BONES & A TOOTH

"The human foot is a masterpiece of engineering and a work of art"
-Leonardo Da Vinci

Hip Joint
8x10 Watercolor
2015

THE GOOD BONES

I see her,
Look closer, dear
I notice her skin,
Explore without fear
I think of tissue below,
Seek still further
Cells working in tandem,
Be a keen observer
Muscle, elegant and strong
Rouse third eye from sleep
Contracting together,
Delve into the deep
Then firm bone,
Beloved, that's it
Her essence buried
Close now, don't quit
I spot her strength,
Yes, my friend
Her rarity, her soul
We are nearing the end
Naught else matters
You can be free
Now that I see
Now that you see
The good bones.

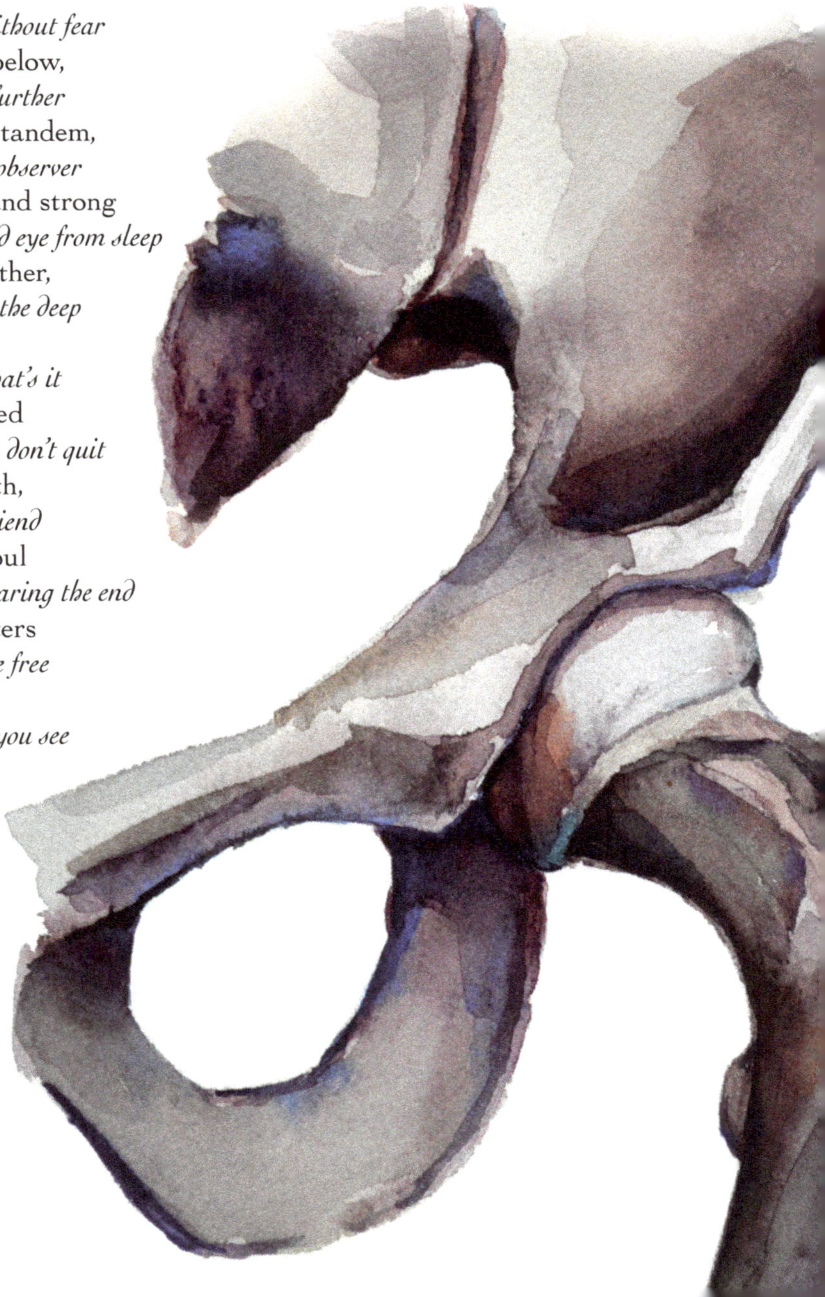

SELLA TURCICA

A Turkish saddle
Sits atop butterfly wings
Cradling gland of life

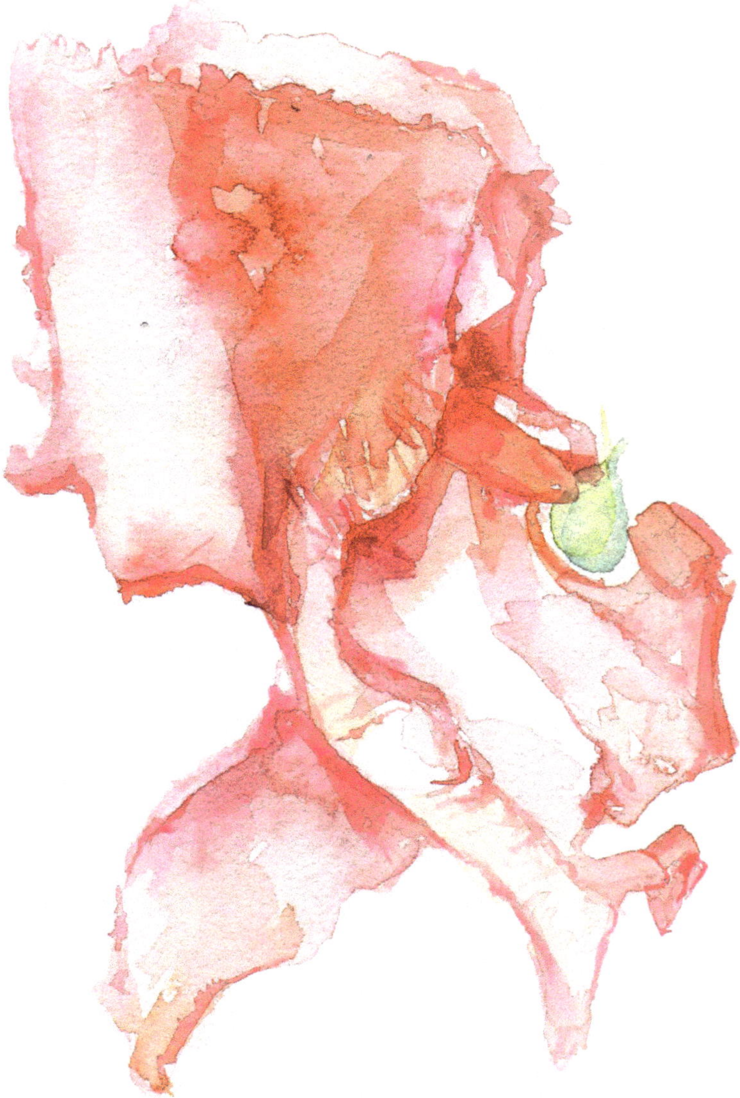

Sphenoid and Pituitary
8x10 Watercolor
2024

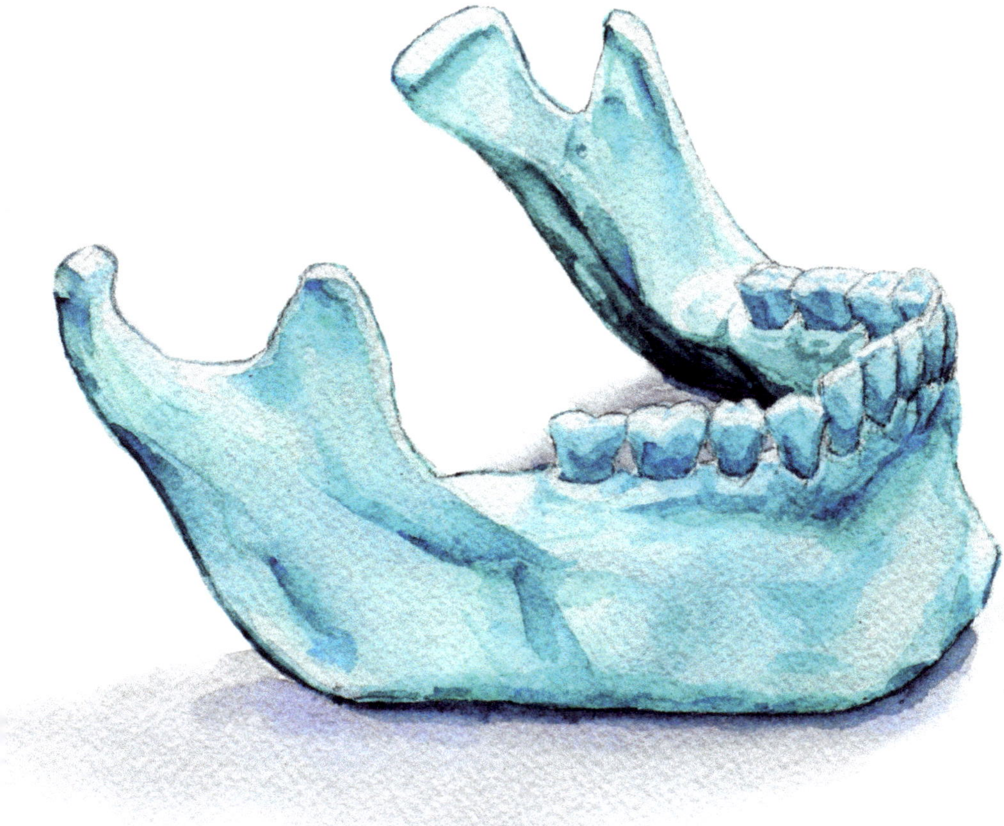

MANDIBLE

Chiseled planes of bone
Weapons of mastication
Sheathed in its chambers

Mandible
8x10 Watercolor
2015

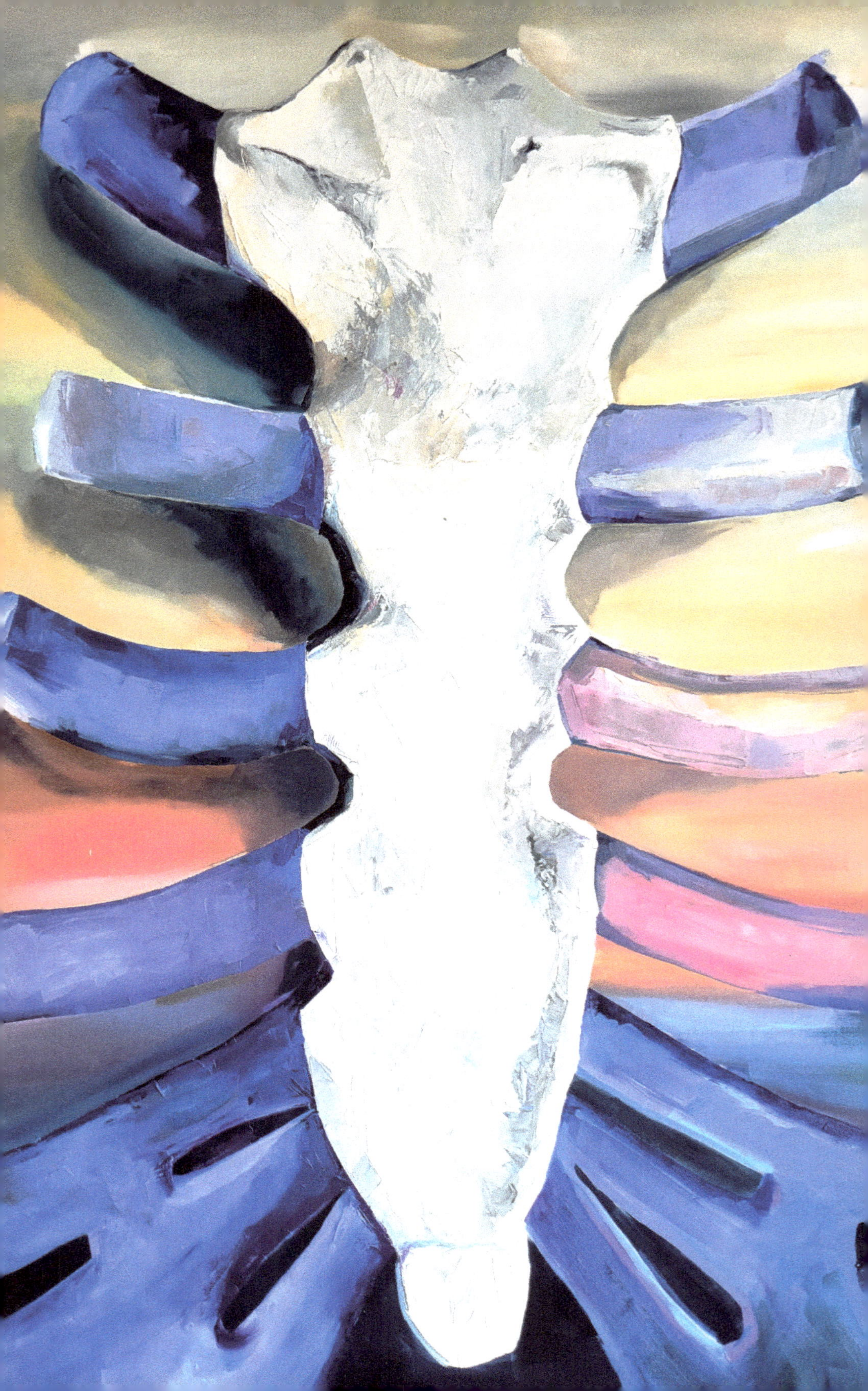

THE PROTECTOR

At our center lies
A shield,
A protector,
A bulwark

Nobly guarding the
Heart beat,
Life pulse,
Soul spark

See its fortitude
And reflect,
Ruminate,
Then hark:

It's time to protect the
Fragile dawn
From an
endless dark.

The Protective Sternum
36x48 Oil on Canvas
2022

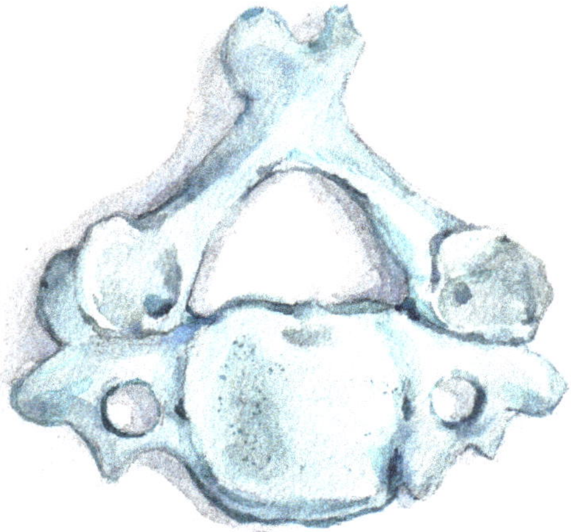

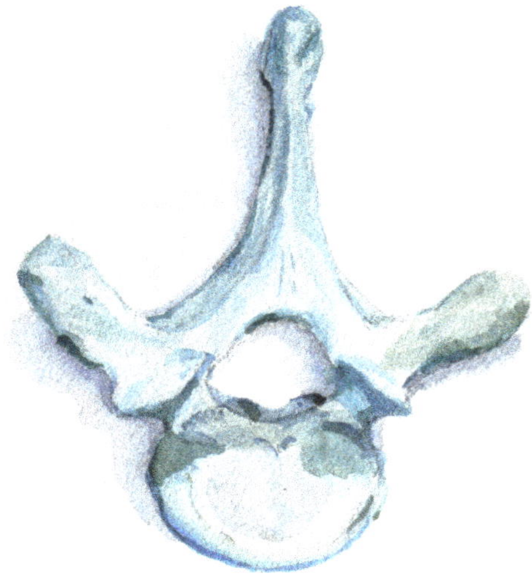

FORKED FANGS

Seven bones in this cervical gang,
Each one with a gnarly forked fang.
It sticks out our back,
makes us unique,
Along with our sleek
three-holed physique.
Our leader is a badass, call him Atlas
He's basically the king of the palace.
He holds up the head all day, no sweat
Though he couldn't
without Axis, I bet—
His number two
who keeps him grounded
Using his dens, big and rounded.
We keep our turf in these upper decks
Controlling all the head and the neck.
Enter our territory at your own risk,
Make us mad and
we'll herniate your disc.

SHARK SPIES

Our thoracic gang
is smooth and cunning.
One look at us twelve
and you'll go running.
For our nasty shark-finned
spinous process
Shows that we don't suffer nonsense.
To a sly rib pair we each attach,
Creating a spy network
that's yet unmatched.
Agent T1 is small and lean.
She can disguise as the cervical team.
T12, too, can go undercover
Faking that she's one of the lumbar.
With this tendency to plot and survey,
And our shifty, sinuous ways
It's no surprise that we hold in our fist
The key to all of the body's twists.

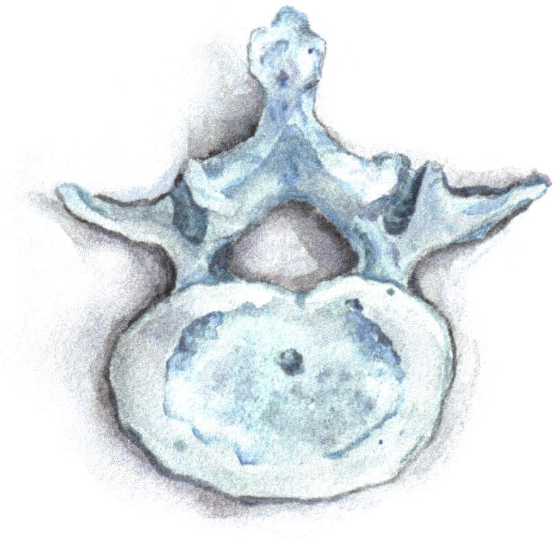

ONE-HORNED OXEN

The other gangs have sleek designs,
More members too,
since we're just five.
But that is way more than enough,
Because like an ox, we are quite tough.
Just picture an ox with one thick horn
Who face their rivals
with naught but scorn.
For while they primp and blow hot air
It's *their* mass we ceaelessly bear.
So if one sly look hits us wrong
We'll make them sing their swan song.
Though to us their bickering
is just nonsense—
We take on much bigger concepts.
Like maintaining a posture
that is straight
And carrying the
WHOLE BODY'S weight!

Cervical Vertebra
8x10 Watercolor
2015

Thoracic Vertebra
8x10 Watercolor
2015

Lumbar Vertebra
8x10 Watercolor
2015

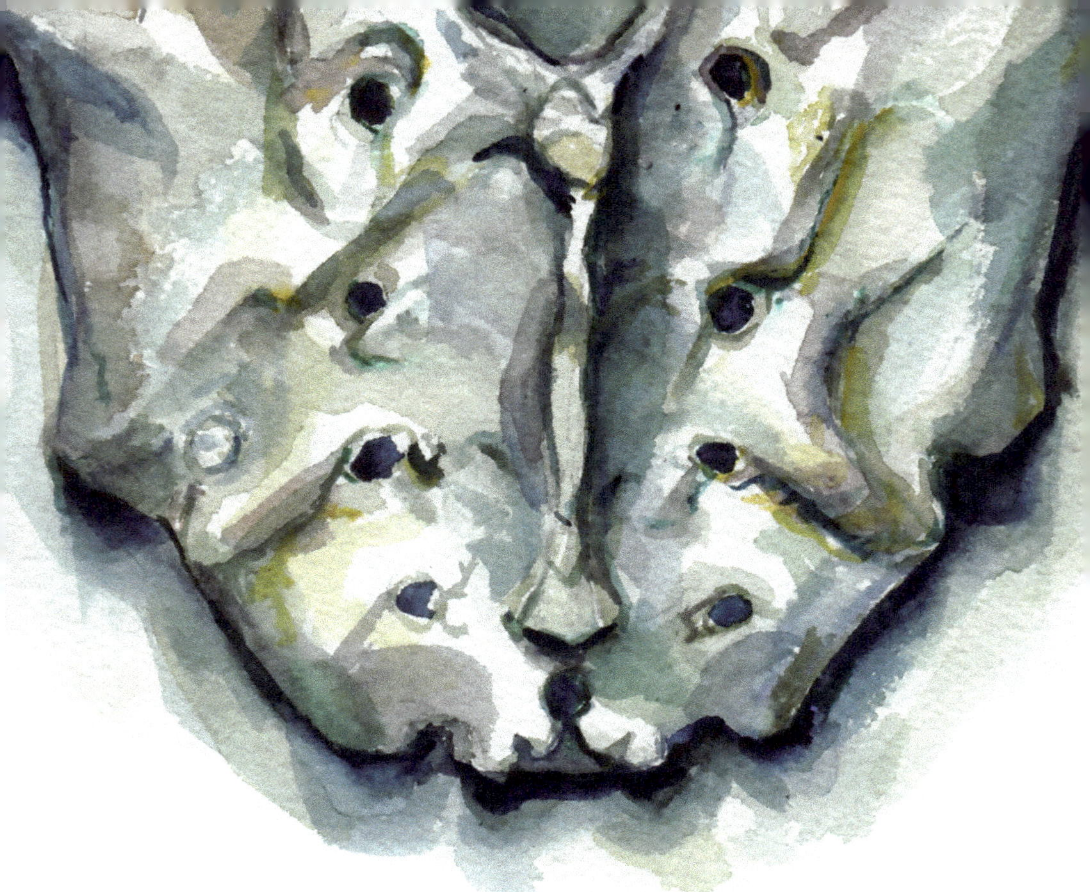

BEHEMOTH

We used to be a gang of five.
But we found it hard to thrive.
Always getting bumped and jostled,
Pushed us into feeling hostile.
The Lumbars claim they bear the weight
When they just move it to our plate.
Then the pelvis says, "Hold steady! Be still!"
Using us against our will.
For years our ire simmered and boiled
As we strained and grunted and toiled.
It seems that anger lent us power
And like magic, we fused into a tower.
Now the others fear to tangle with
A two-horned, eight-eyed sacral behemoth.

Sacrum
8x10 Watercolor
2022

HURT FEELINGS

Since we no longer have a tail
My presence is a little stale.
I have, though, picked up a side hustle
As an attachment point for some muscles.
Indeed, without me the pelvic floor
Wouldn't be functional anymore.
Despite this, I find my reputation
Is based on just one situation.
See, I'm the one who gets mauled
When you take a bottom-first fall.
And I know I cause pain like the thrust
Of a thousand knives up your butt.
But please don't curse me when you're reeling.
Because I'm not pointless, and I do have feelings.

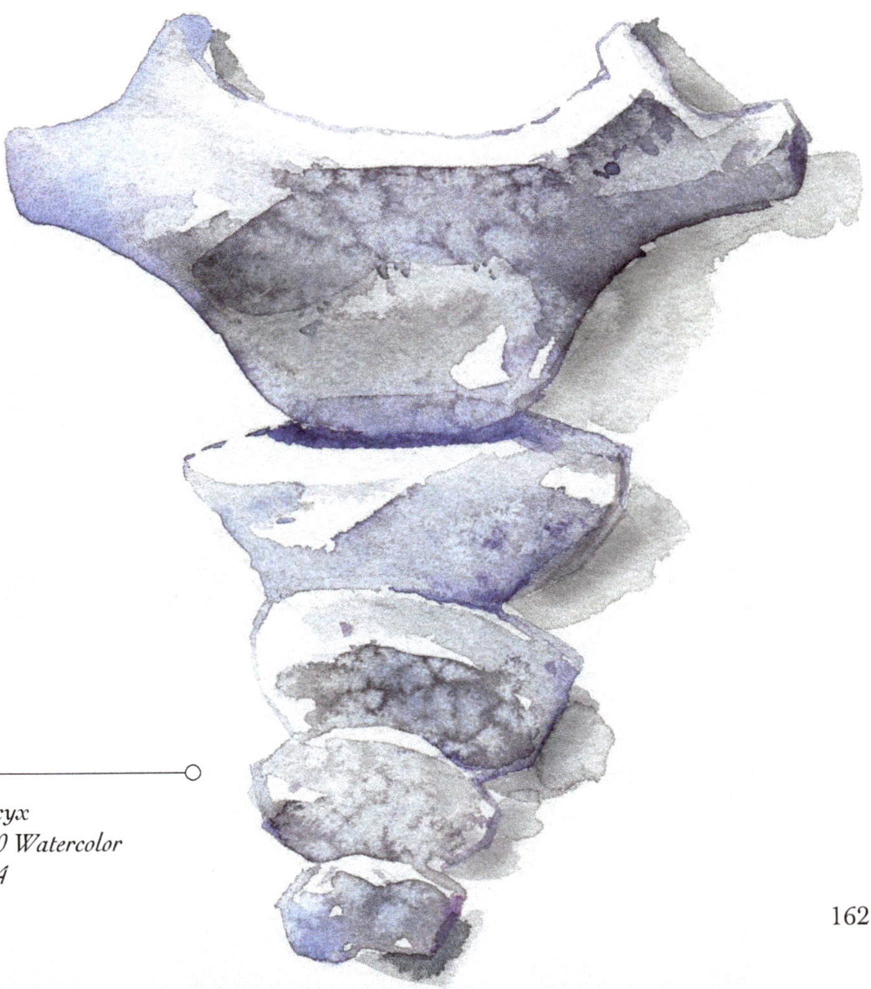

Coccyx
8x10 Watercolor
2024

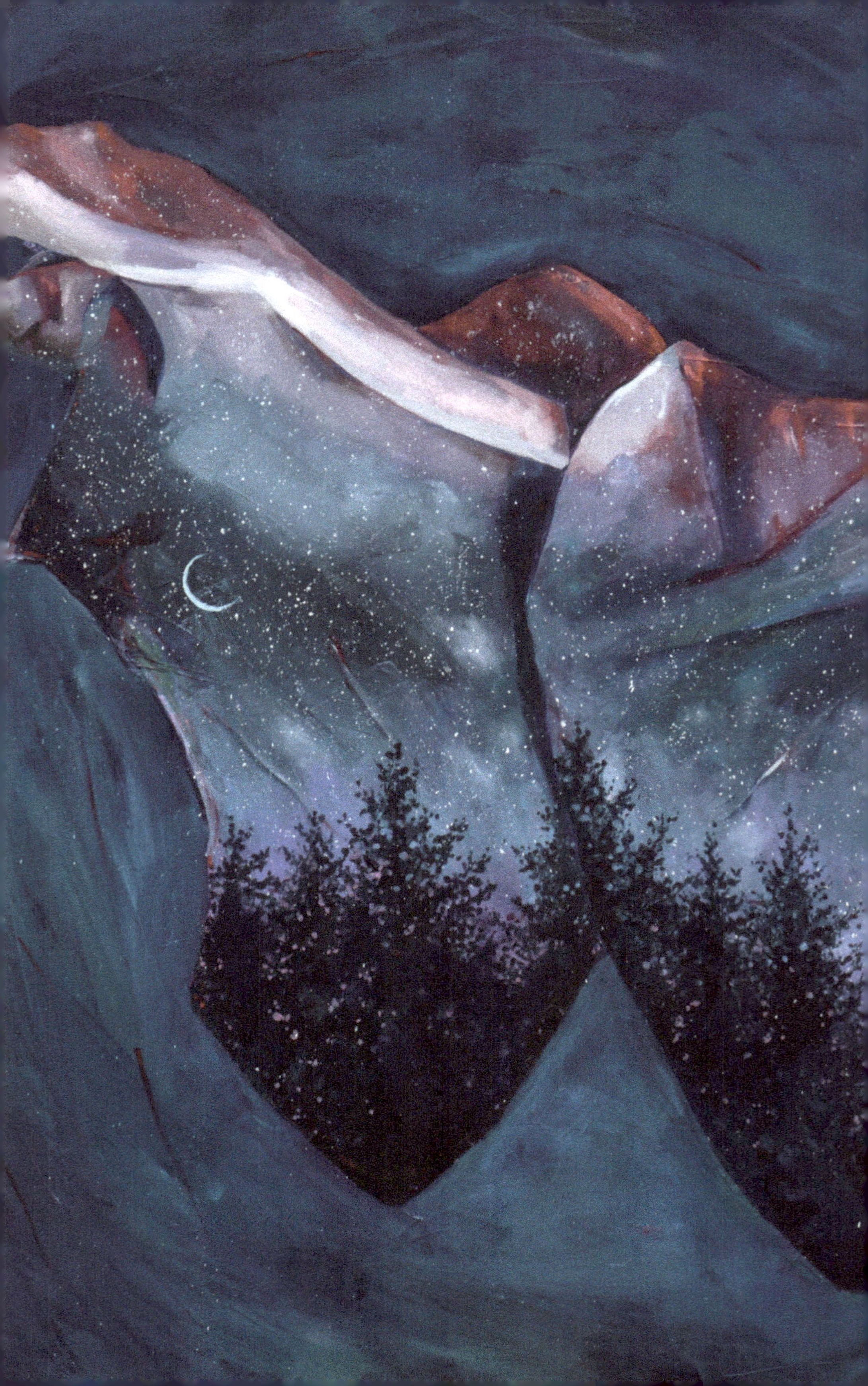

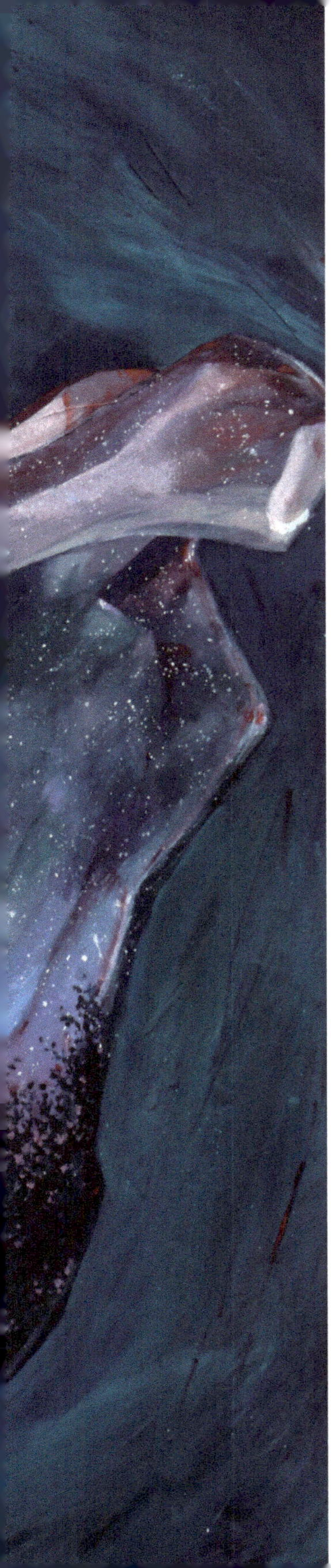

WORLD ON MY SHOULDERS

Child, you are my world.
The world rests on my shoulders.
A burden, of love.

World on My Shoulders
36x36 Oil on Canvas
2023

HAND OF THE KING

In the great Land of the Body, King Brain has the throne,
Ruling each province with care, joy and skill.
But he can't enforce his decisions alone,
So who does he trust to impose his will?

The Hand of the King! The Hand of the King!
The great executor of the brain's every whim!
To him let us sing! To him let us sing!
He who does the handling, no matter how grim!

Little did you know that the Hand of the King
Is made up of courtiers, so skillful and brave.
Nineteen members that endlessly bring
Agility so we can grasp, grip and wave.

So... to the Court of the Hand! The Court of the Hand!
A bony, royal assemblage that brings prosperity!
For you do we stand! For you do we stand!
We love you with the deepest sincerity!

Five Metacarpal Dukes abide in the palm,
Five Proximal Phalanges have been honored as earls.
Four Viscount Middle Phalanges are known for their calm,
The five Distal Phalange Barons can curl and unfurl.

So... to the Bones of the Court! The Bones of the Court
Never has there been such nimble nobility!
It's you we support! It's you we support!
We have you to thank for our endless abilities!

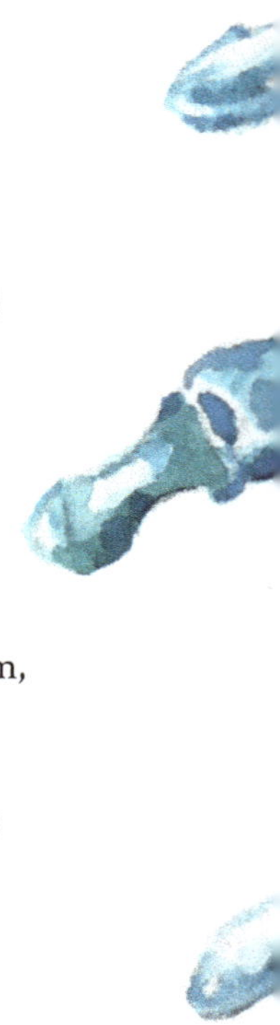

Hand Bones
8x10 Watercolor
2015

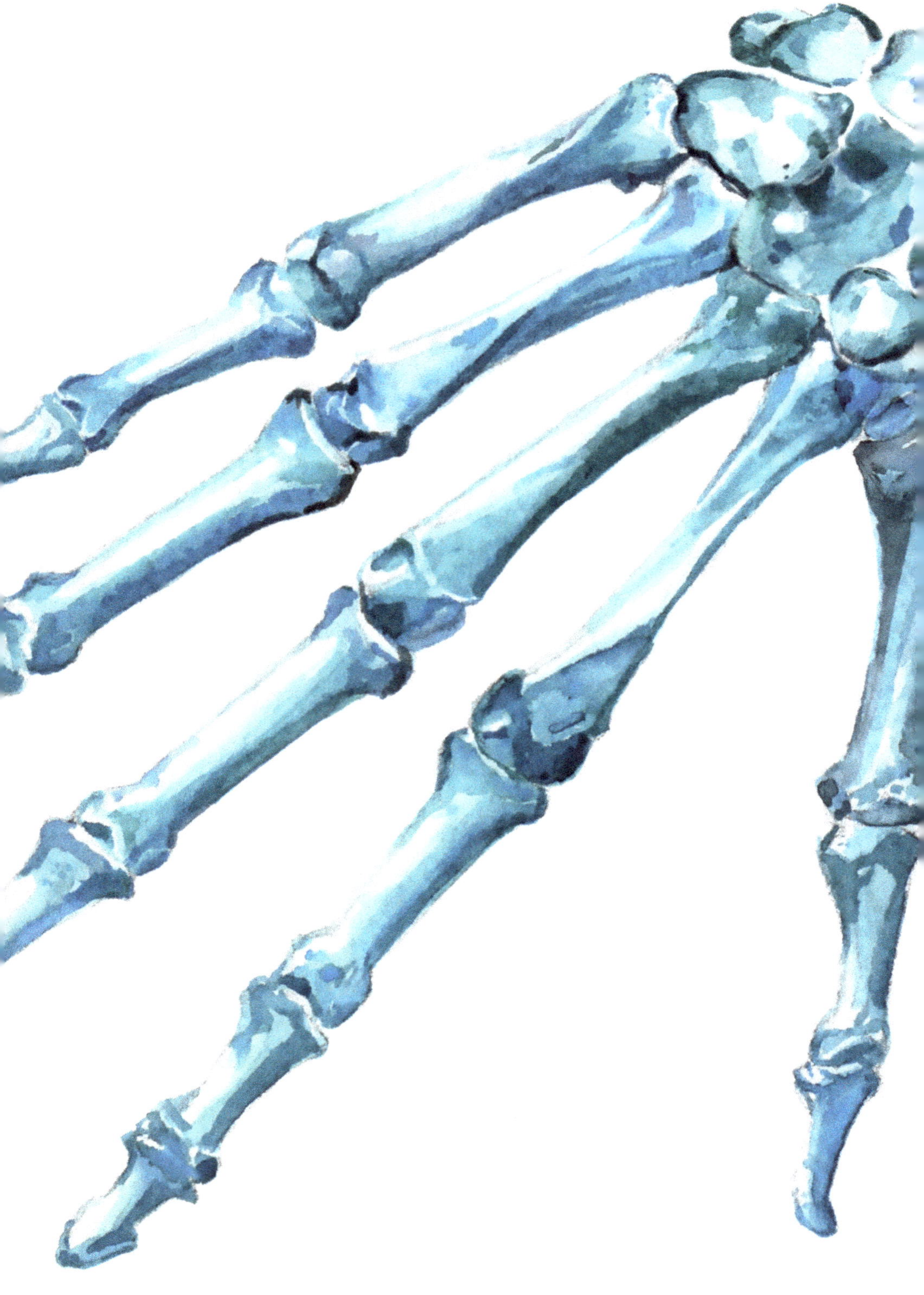

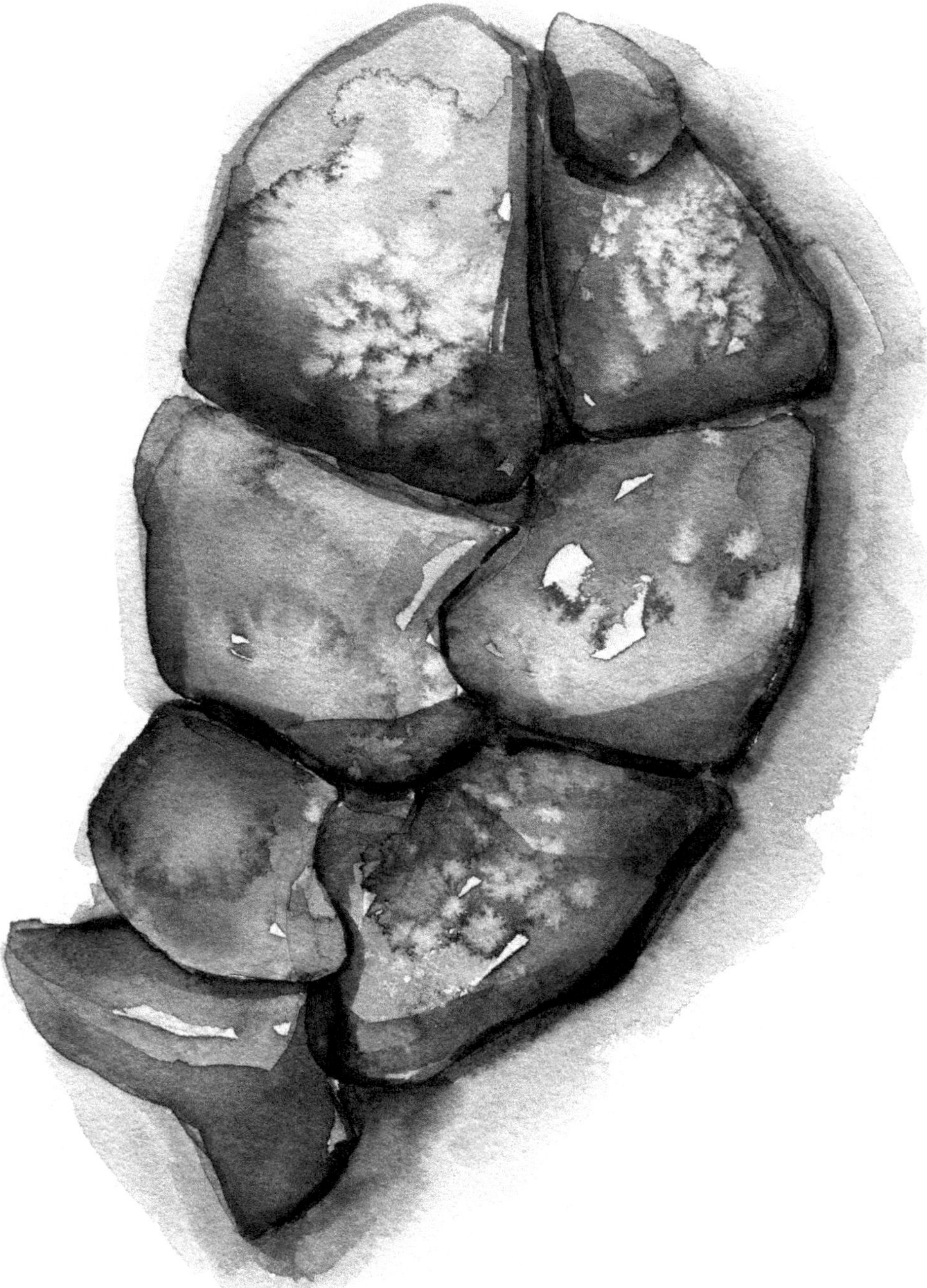

THE STAFF

The royal courtiers of the Noble Hand
Need endless support as they rule the land.

Fortunately, some servants abide in the wrist
So just sit back while I give you the list.

At the base of the thumb is the head of the staff,
The Butler Trapezium, who never laughs.

His right-hand woman is the housekeeper:
Ms. Trapezoid, in charge of the sweepers.

Next is the valet, a Mr. Capitate
(His rival is Butler, whom he really hates.)

The last of the upper staff is Mrs. Hamate,
The best lady's maid in the whole estate.

Scaphoid is a footman with a deep Irish brogue
Low on the hierarchy, but a handsome rogue!

Nearby the two housemaids both crush on him:
Triquetum and Lunate, both sweet but dim.

Last of the group is the small scullery maid,
Wee pisiform; hardest worker, smallest paid.

Thanks to the toil of this diligent group,
The Noble Hand can bend, twist, flex and scoop.

Bones of the Wrist
8x10 Watercolor
2024

THE RESILIENT PELVIS

Buried deep, a lowly basin
Cradles a seed of untold wealth.
The pelvis, site of transformation
Of my child, of myself.

Life is forged, life unfurls
Life bulldozes its way out
In its path, leaving a whirl
Of love and joy, pain and doubt.

As my mind and bones resettle,
I grasp that life comes with a cost.
I thought that I had mettle,
Yet I'm now different, alone and lost.

But just as aspen after a fire
Is first to rise among the cinders,
So will I conquer this mire,
A small, brave bud outlasting winter.

Buried deep, a lowly basin
Is bent and beat, then reforms.
Now I know, without hesitation,
That I can withstand any storm.

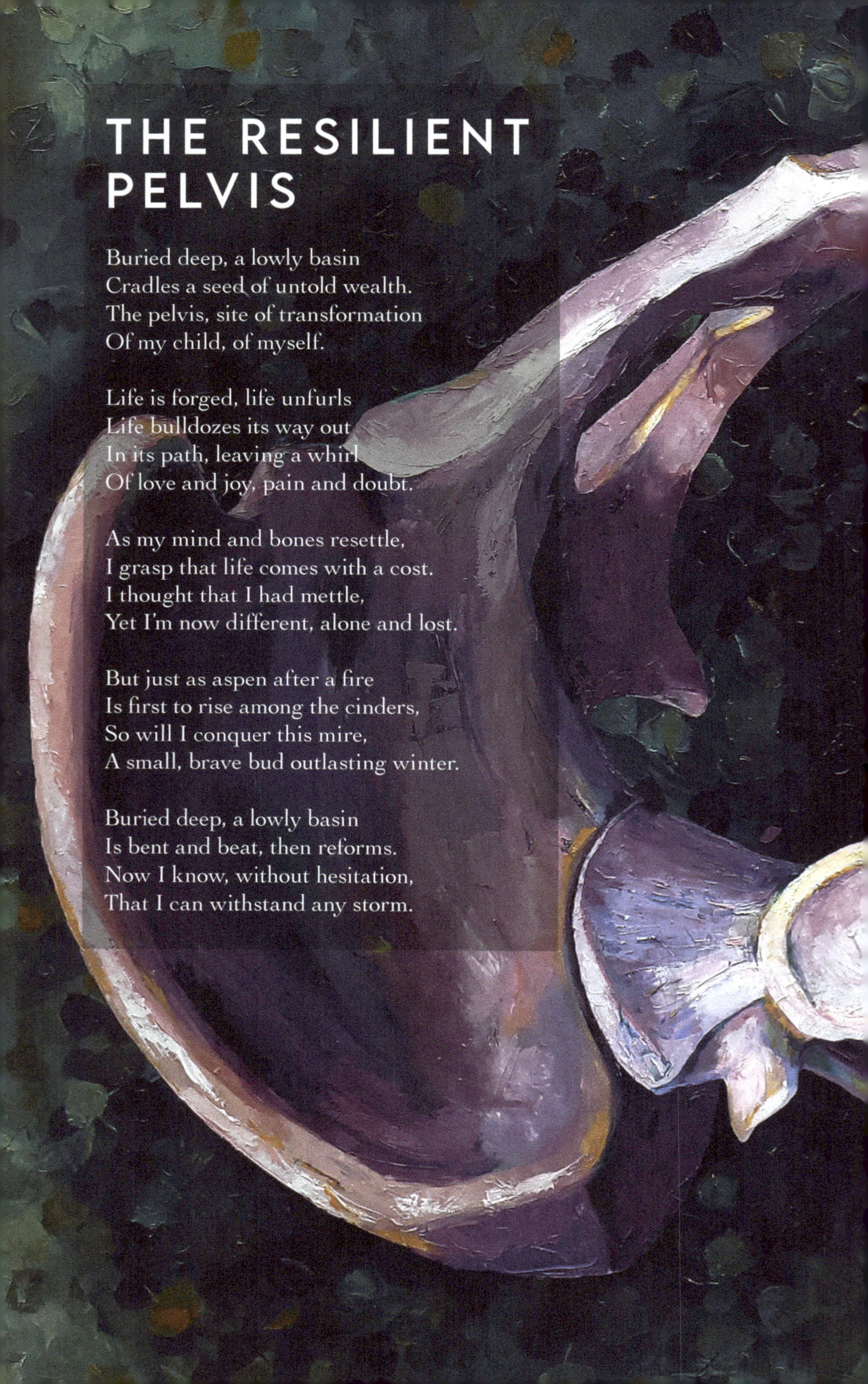

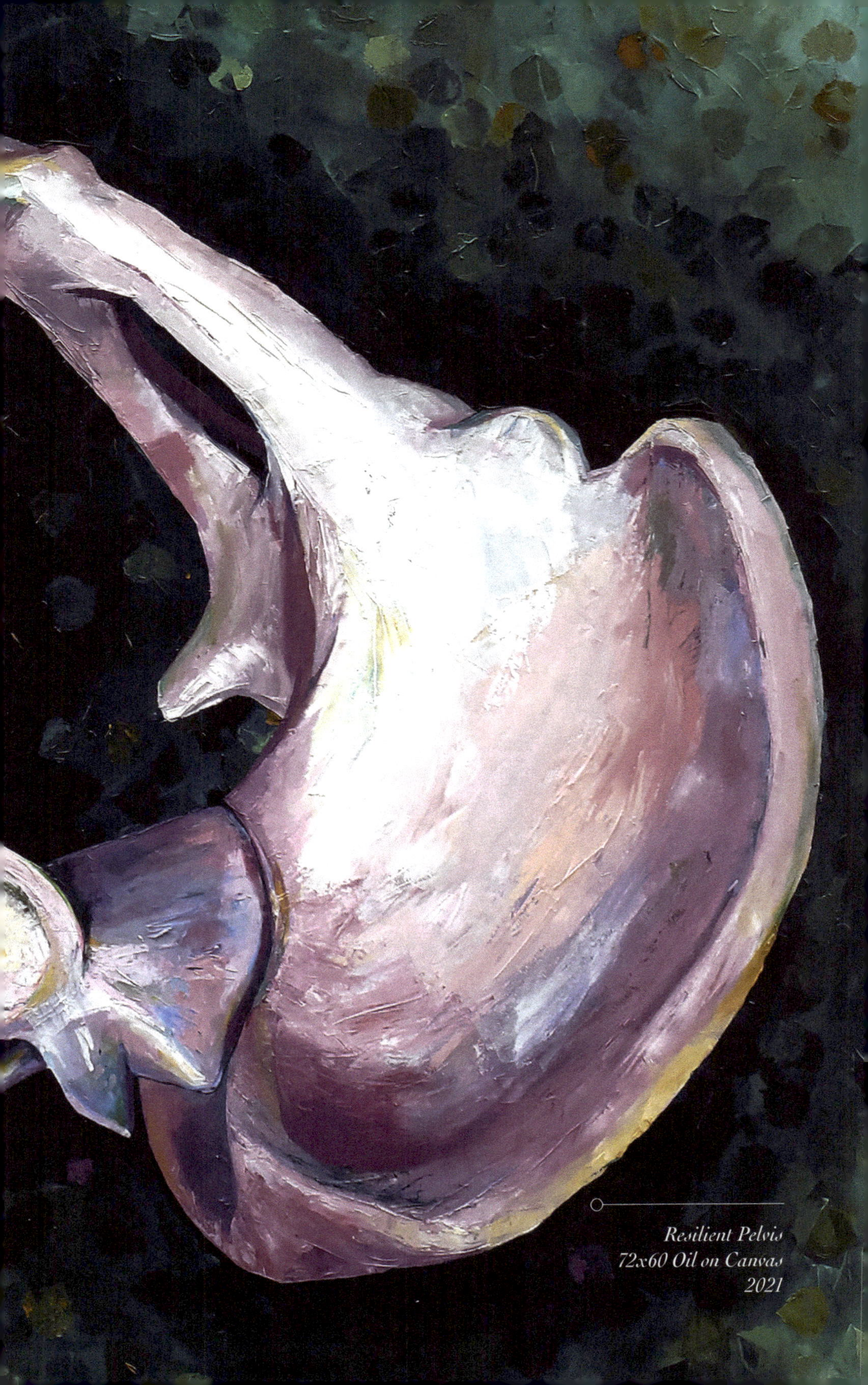

Resilient Pelvis
72x60 Oil on Canvas
2021

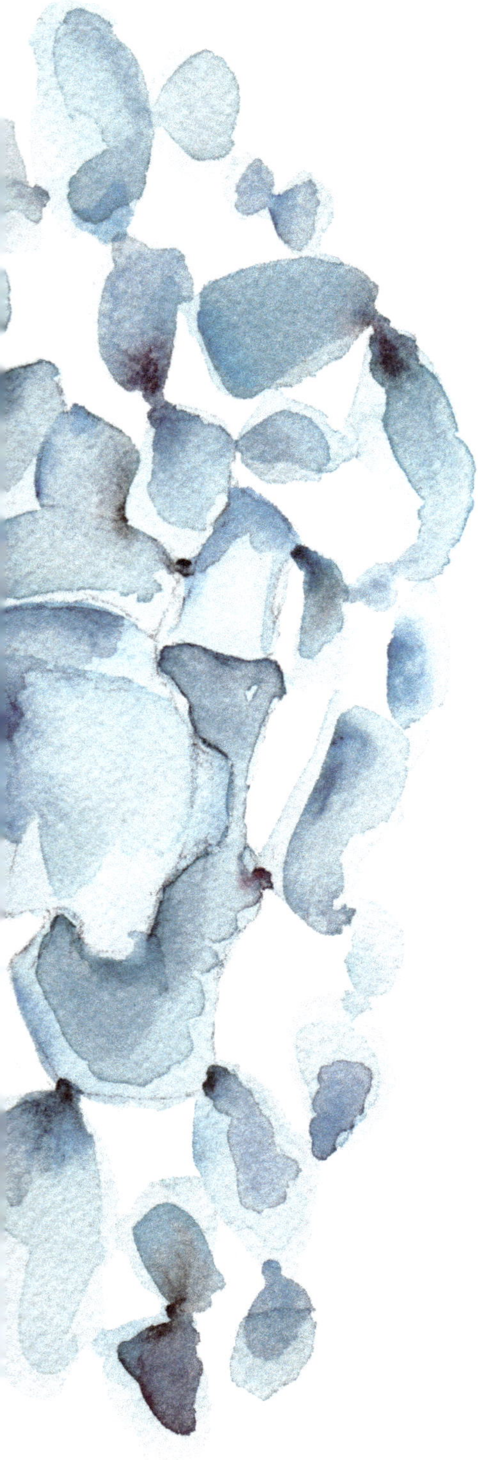

MIDNIGHT LAUNDRY

For my mom

It was the middle of the night
When she woke up in a fright.
She felt an internal quandary,
For did she ever switch the laundry?
She thought it best just to check,
Really, it would only take a sec,
And damp clothes with smells detectable
Would be simply unacceptable.
Tiptoeing her way down the hall,
Feeling carefully along the wall,
Though darkness was a curtain,
Her walk became more certain.
"One more step until the stair!"
She thought with a confident flair.
So one more stride she took,
Without even taking a look.
Into thin air she stumbled,
Head over heels as she tumbled.
Landing in a painful heap,
Her right foot hurting deep.
She knew it was more than a callous—
Turns out she had broke her talus.
With weeks until recovery,
She made an important discovery
Midnight laundry inventory
Isn't really worth the glory.

Hidden Tarsal Bones
8x10 Watercolor
2015

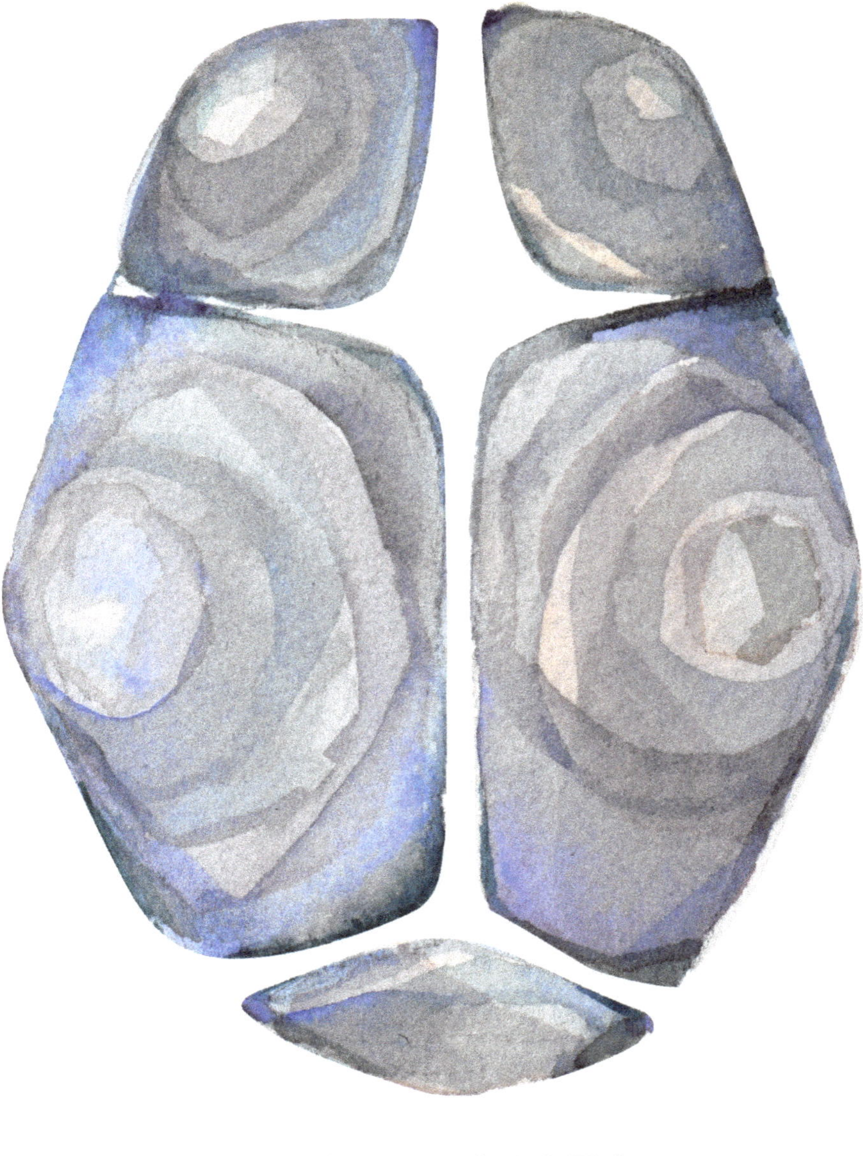

FONTANEL

Four bones' unstitched seams
Form a velvety hollow.
Keep the gateway safe.

Fontanel
8x10 Watercolor
2015

A LOVE HEPTAGON

Some say a love triangle's bound to cause pain,
Drama that only goes wrong.
To us orbital bones, that all seems mundane—
Compared to our love heptagon.

We blame our suggestive behavior on just
A simple lack of real estate
There's four small rooms but seven of us
So we are forced to all cohabitate.

Sweet frontal lives with sphenoid up top
In a penthouse a bit monotonous.
You may think that couple's strong, but they're not.
Since just one of them's monogamous.

For Sphenoid also shares a bed
in the lateral apartment.
And gets naughty with Zygoma, it's said,
Within that small compartment.

But there's more we feel we must expose
Of Sphenoid's dirty deeds:
For across the lot he sneakily goes
To sow his wildest seeds.

To a naughty, wicked place of lust
Known as the Medial Wall
Here you'll scope fine Ethmoid's bust
And almost all of Lacrimal.

Even so, we think it's Maxillary
That keeps Sphenoid staying inside.
For a secret love's been burning very
deep within his mind.

Now Maxillary owns a second place
A bit more respectable.
She has a key to the basement space
Where she is less of a spectacle.

Her roommates there are Palatine
And Zygoma, remember her?
She's also the one who got entwined,
With Sphenoid, that roving cur.

His passion toward her seems overacted,
Just a bit overzealous.
We think it's just a plan he's enacted
To make Maxillary jealous!

This love heptagon creates a tapestry
Of lechery, love and lies.
Housing hope and tragedy
Along with both the eyes!

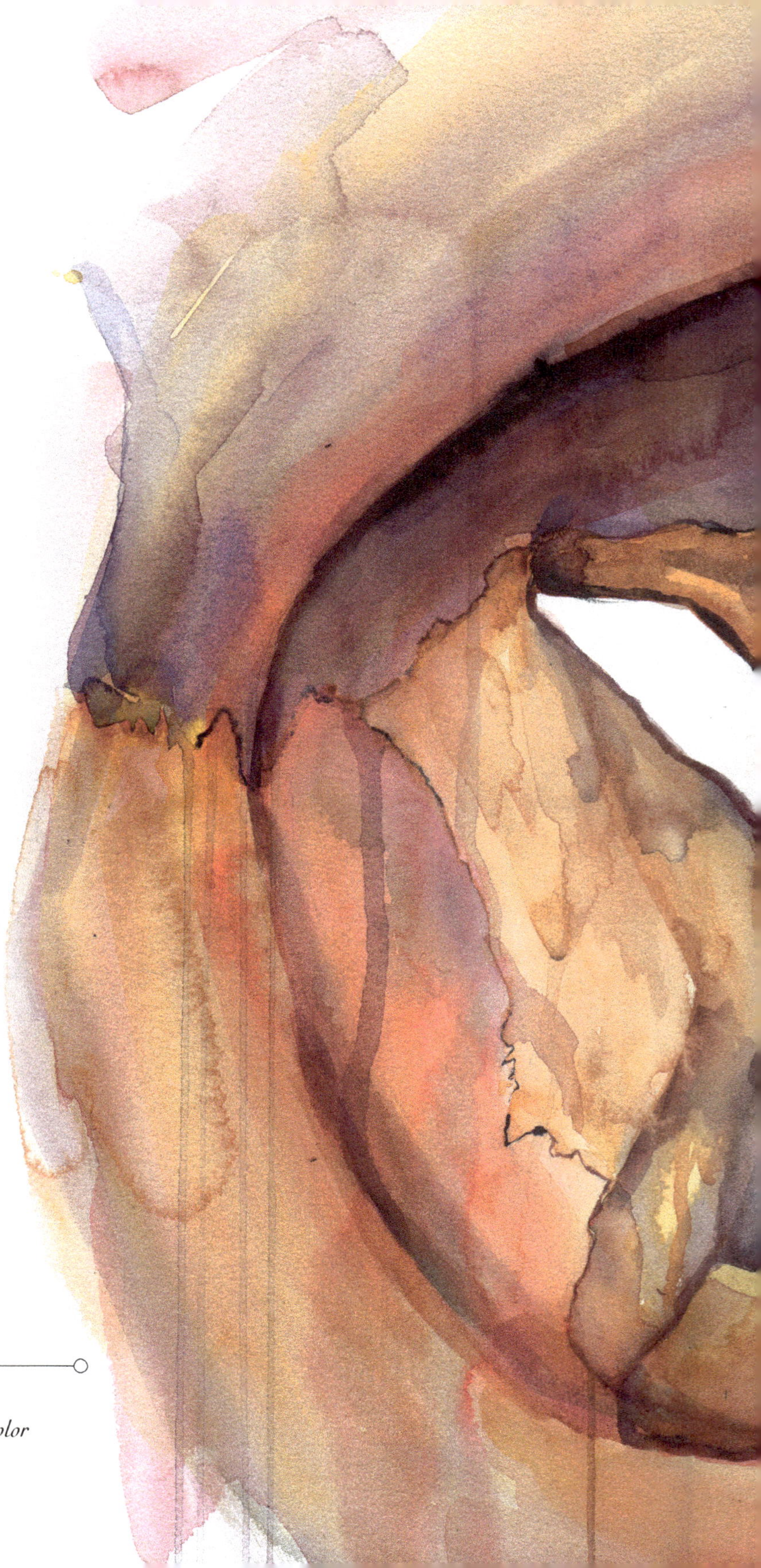

The Orbit
22x22 Watercolor
2024

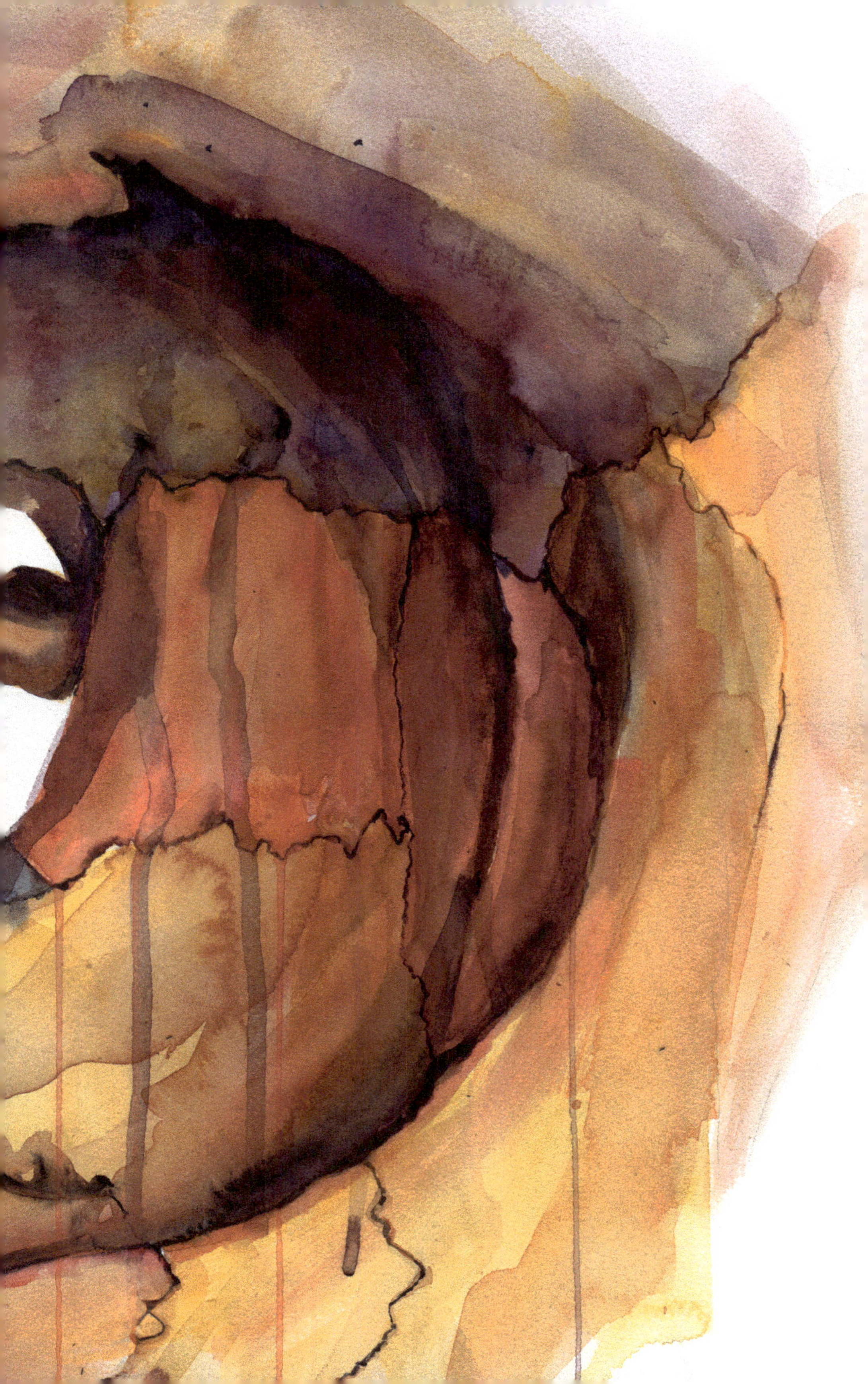

TIBIAL TUBEROSITY

Roughened hill of bone
Kisses patella's white rope
The leg can stretch now

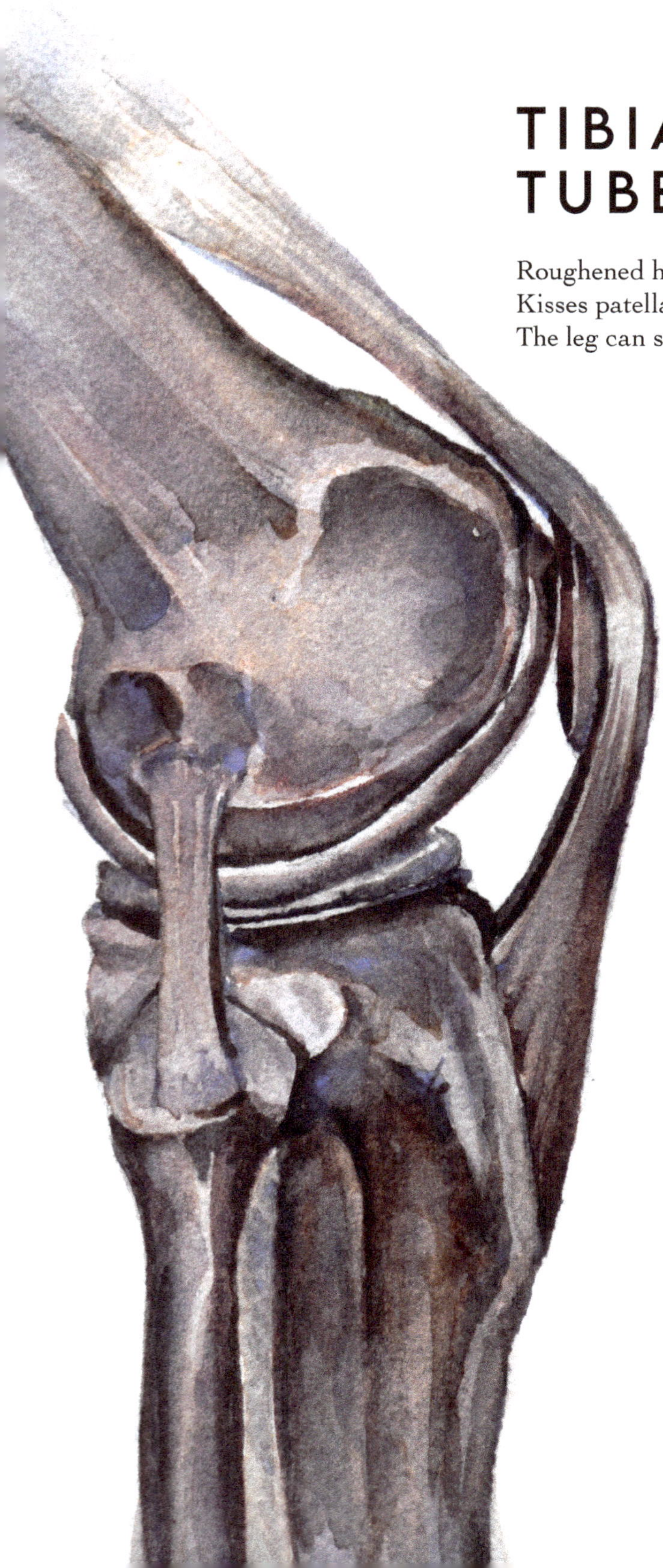

Knee Joint
8x10 Watercolor
2015

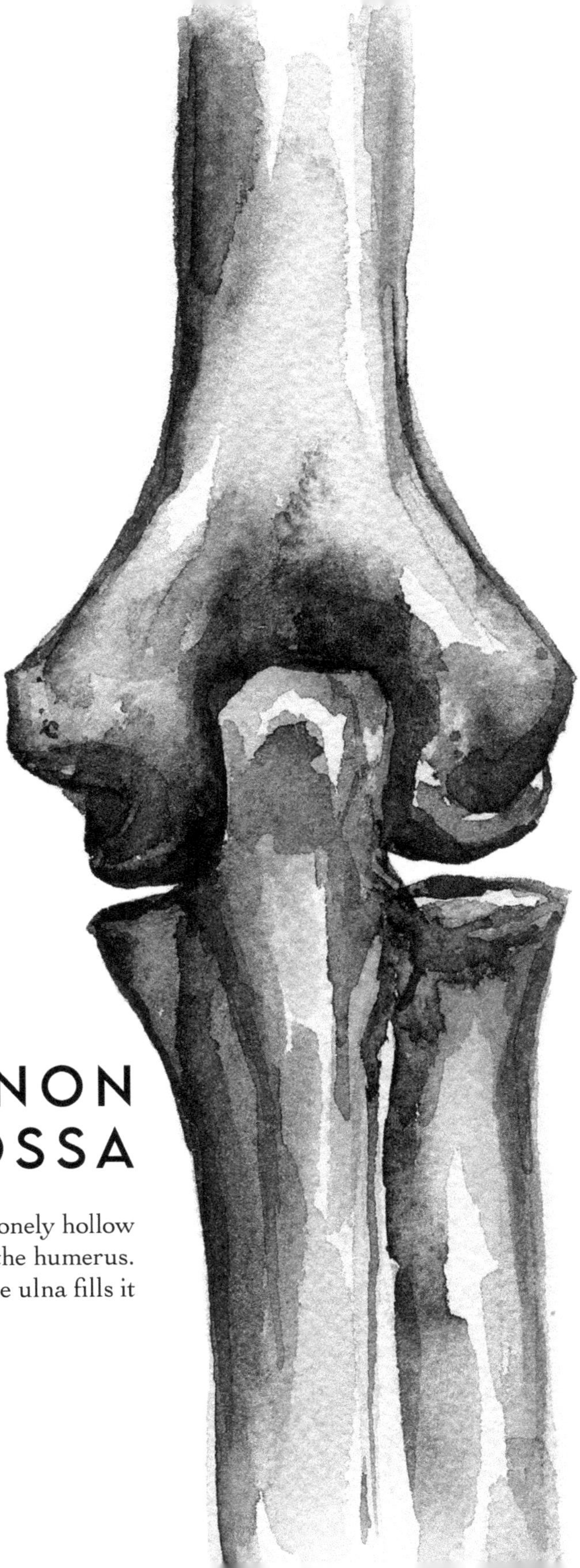

OLECRANON FOSSA

A lonely hollow
Lurks behind the humerus.
The ulna fills it

Elbow Joint
8x10 Watercolor
2018

THE BALLAD OF CARABELLI

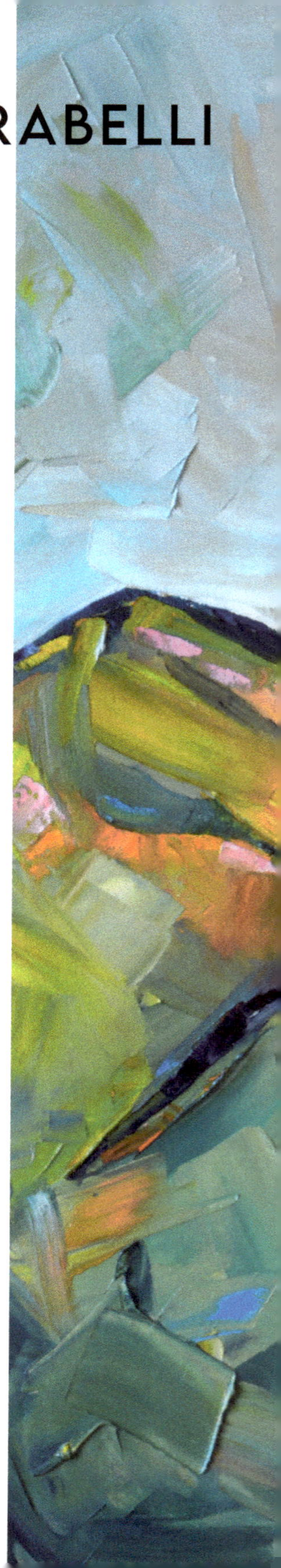

I traverse along these bluffs of luster,
In search of a fabled peak.
Nestled among these pearly clusters,
A milky-white sculpture I seek.
Climbers like me, who are far from meek
On a quest to mount the belly
Of a cliff that weeds out the weak,
I hunt the Cusp Carabelli.

A place where fear will be castigated—
Though I know the terrain be daunting,
And any frailty must be masticated—
Though that outcropping can be haunting.
Many mouths I've plundered but alas, left wanting,
No mound to be found in that valley.
The ache to prove my worth still taunting,
I'll find that Cusp Carabelli.

What if this structure has all been a myth?
Is my life's crusade just for show?
But wait—just there—rising out of the fifth
Dental edifice within this row—
I have finally found my mountainous foe!
I traverse pink terrain on legs of jelly,
And at last under that crag, I know...
I fear the Cusp Carabelli.

I might fall, I might perish, this risk is needless!
Then again... what if I survive?
What if I scale the impossible, heedless
Of doubts about staying alive?
Can I surpass my fears and take the dive?
It may sound quite Machiavelli,
But the means are worth it, in order to thrive.
I'll scale the Cusp Carabelli.

Painstakingly I climb, my brow in a furrow
Near the top, I start to feel heavy.
But lo, I've made it! I now can just burrow.
Bacteria's found home on Cusp Carabelli!

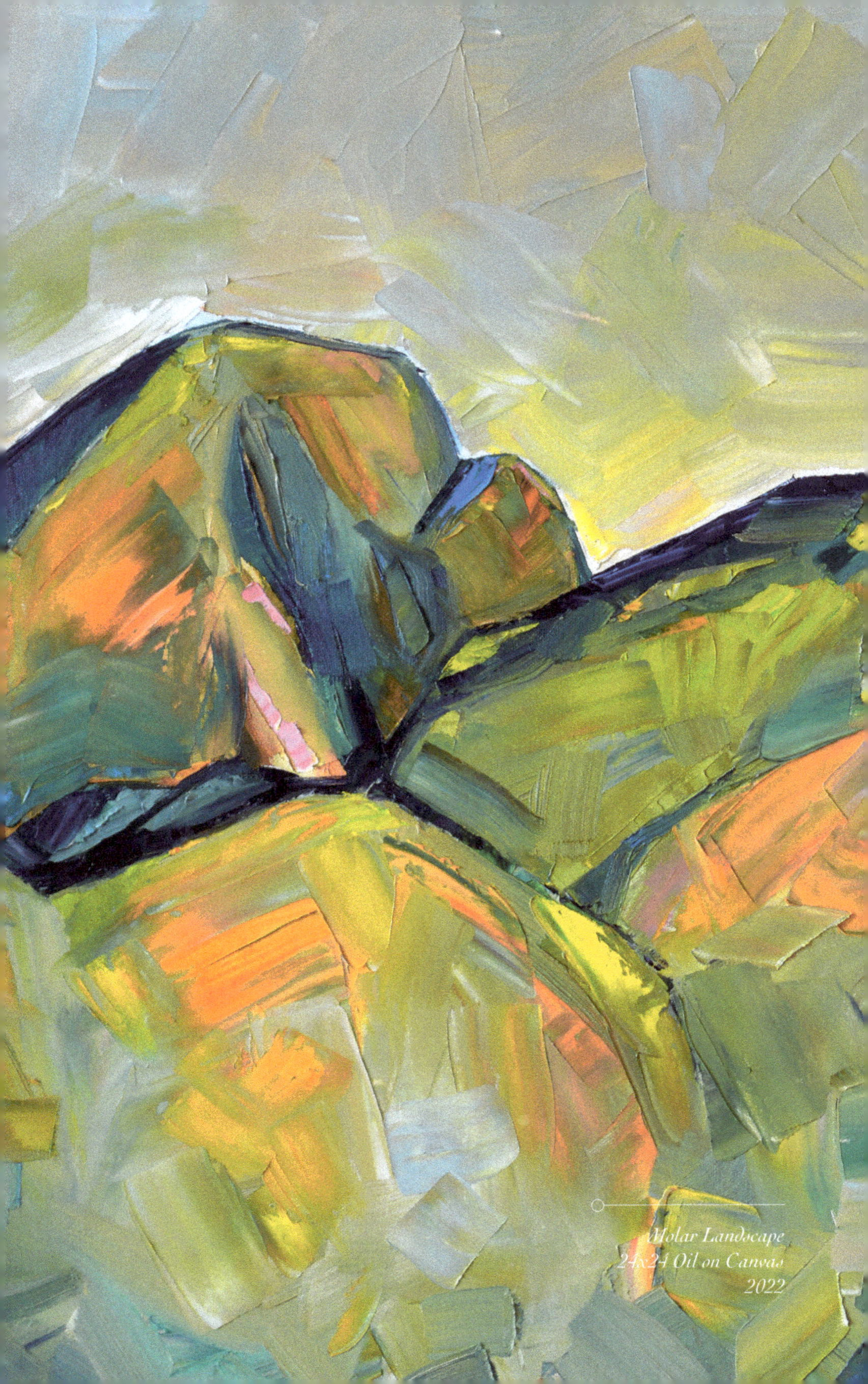

Molar Landscape
24x24 Oil on Canvas
2022

INDEX OF PAINTINGS

INDEX OF POEMS

GENERAL INDEX

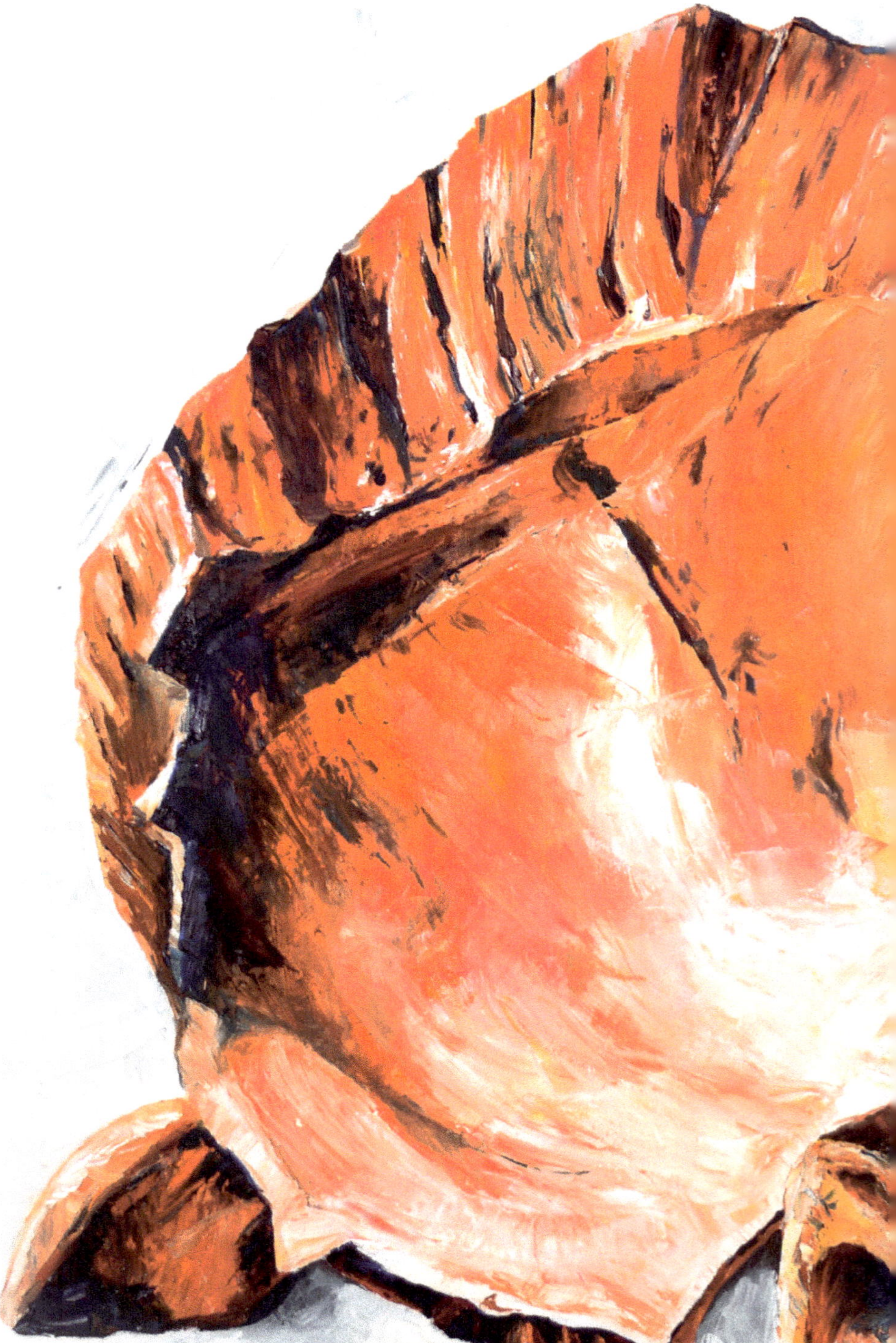

Temporal Bone
48x36 Oil on Canvas
2018

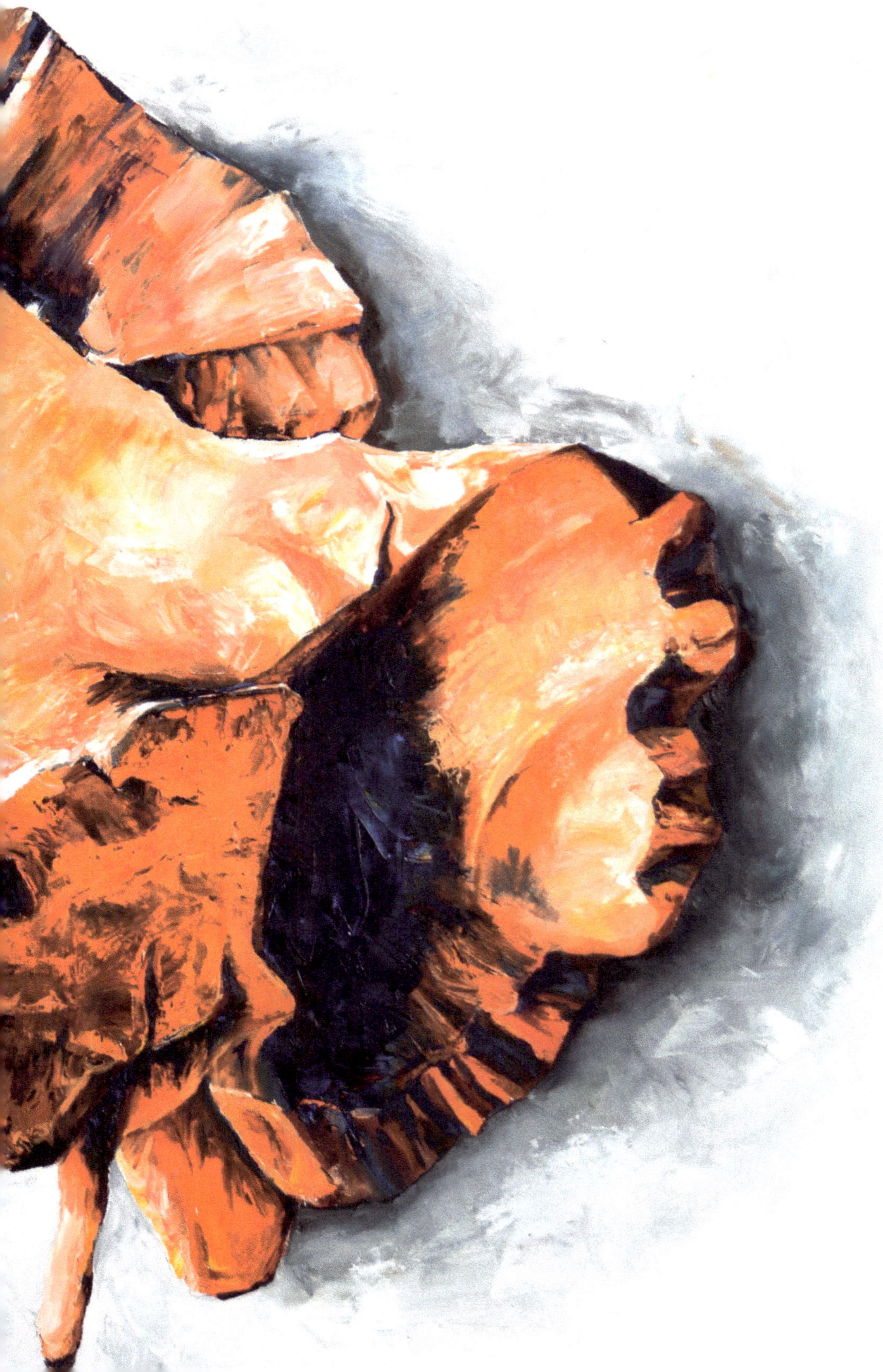

www.ingramcontent.com/pod-product-compliance
Lightning Source LLC
LaVergne TN
LVHW051055210926
848486LV00002B/117
9798218389468